ATLAS OF

BREAST CANCER

merit

PUBLISHING
INTERNATIONAL

ATLAS OF
BREAST CANCER

ROGER BLAMEY
PROFESSOR OF SURGICAL SCIENCE · NOTTINGHAM CITY HOSPITAL

ANDREW EVANS
CONSULTANT RADIOLOGIST · NOTTINGHAM CITY HOSPITAL

IAN ELLIS
CONSULTANT HISTOPATHOLOGIST · NOTTINGHAM CITY HOSPITAL

ROBIN WILSON
CONSULTANT RADIOLOGIST · NOTTINGHAM CITY HOSPITAL

merit
PUBLISHING
INTERNATIONAL

PROVIDED AS A SERVICE TO MEDICAL EDUCATION BY

ZENECA Pharma.

ATLAS OF
BREAST CANCER

PUBLISHED BY:
MERIT PUBLISHING INTERNATIONAL

USA address :

8260 N.W. 49th Manor,
Pine Grove, Coral Springs,
Florida 33067
U.S.A.

European address :

35 Winchester Street,
Basingstoke,
Hampshire, RG21 1EE,
U.K.

ISBN: 1 873413 70 X

Printed by Butler & Tanner Ltd, Frome and London

merit
PUBLISHING
INTERNATIONAL

CONTENTS

FOREWORD

ALEXANDER J. WALT, DISTINGUISHED PROFESSOR OF SURGERY,
WAYNE STATE UNIVERSITY, DETROIT, MICHIGAN.

The incidence of breast cancer in the industrialized world has increased alarmingly over recent decades. In parallel, diagnosis and clinical management have become bewilderingly complex. The past 20 years have seen the demise of biopsy and immediate resolution by radical mastectomy in a single intellectually unchallenging and socially insensitive operation. Today, mammography, ultrasonography, fine needle aspiration and stereotactic core biopsy have come of age. Surgical operations are now tailored to the biology of the lesion while adjunctive irradiation, chemotherapy, and hormonal manipulations are harnessed in the pursuit of improved results.

Examiners of candidates seeking higher surgical degrees often have difficulty in agreeing on the appropriate answers to their constantly expanding questions, which now include considerations of genetic analysis and counselling, the natural history of in situ carcinomas, the significance and hierarchy of prognostic factors, the value of flow cytometry and tumor markers, and a proliferating host of biological measurements.

In the midst of this sophisticated chaos, the Nottingham Breast Centre, led by Professor Roger Blamey, has been a beacon of common sense. In this concise and practical monograph, we are reminded again that in the beginning there is always a patient with a history, physical signs, and a mammogram. The importance of these as the foundation of practical planning is properly stressed and placed in broad perspective. Arguments are backed up by data and descriptions by instructive pictures. This refreshing approach is reminiscent of Zachary Cope's slim monograph on 'The Acute Abdomen,' which has remained a classic for almost seventy years and continues to guide grateful readers across the world. The breast has deserved a similar succinct primer for all family physicians and clinicians who examine the breasts of patients and who seek a broad framework for their observations. It now has one.

SECTION 1

A REVIEW OF BREAST CANCER

SECTION 1

THE DIAGNOSTIC CLINIC

Patients are referred by their family doctors to breast clinics for a variety of reasons (Table 1). The most usual is that the patient believes she may have a breast lump. Other common reasons are breast pain and nipple symptoms (in-drawing, discharge or soreness).

Skill and experience in examination of the breast are essential.

Inspection

The physical signs to look for are *Lump* (Figure 1), *Inflammation* (Figures 2 & 3), *and Tether* (Figures 4,5&6). This sequence is easily remembered in mnemonic form by substituting the word 'Tumor' for 'Lump'!

1. The patient sits on the edge of the couch facing the examiner, who stands directly in front.

2. The patient raises her arms slowly and places them behind her head (Figure 7).

Palpation

Prop the patient up to around 30 degrees (Figure 8). Palpate with the flat of the fingers (Figure 9), never pick up the tissue between the fingers. Palpate with the woman's arms by her side, then with her hands on her head and finally with the patient sitting up and leaning forward a little.

If the lump cannot be felt, ask the patient to put one finger on it: this is a useful guide - if she goes straight to it with one finger then there is a true lump. If she feels vaguely around or picks up the breast tissue between her fingers, then there is no true lump.

Decide which of the following circumstances apply before carrying out investigations:
1. A true lump or other abnormality such as nipple eczema is present. This requires a final diagnosis, the need for which is not changed by imaging.
2. The breasts are normal.
3. There is no definite abnormality but the examiner remains a little uncertain about, for example, a lumpy area with no true lump. Reassessment, either by imaging or by re-examination at a different time of the menstrual cycle, is advised.

LUMPS

The overwhelming majority of true lumps are cysts, fibroadenomas or carcinomas.

Lump in breast	933
Tender 'lumpy' area	110
Breast pain	224
Nipple discharge	75
Nipple retraction	36
Nipple eczema	3
Swelling of breast	7
Others	57
	——
TOTAL	1445

Table 1

The symptoms of 1445 consecutive cases referred to a specialized breast clinic. Belief by the patient that she has a lump in the breast is much the most common symptom, followed by breast pain. Breast pain without the presence of a palpable lump is not a symptom of breast cancer and is a common benign problem.

Figure 1

Lump. A lump is clearly seen on inspection of the left breast.

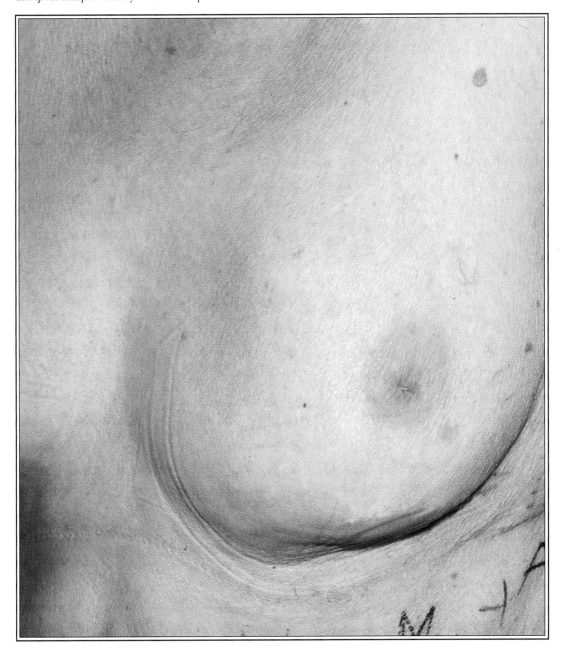

Figure 2

Inflammation. An inflamed area due to an abscess in the breast is easily seen.

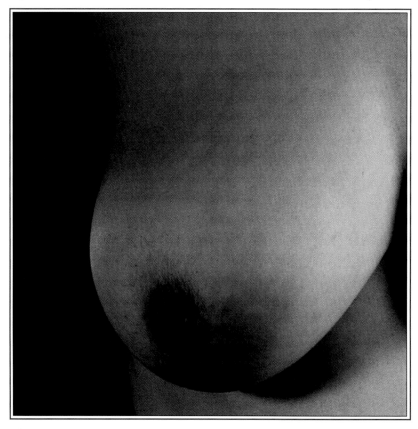

Figure 3

Inflammation of the nipple. The considerable area of excoriation of the nipple and areola seen in this case is caused by Paget's disease of the nipple.

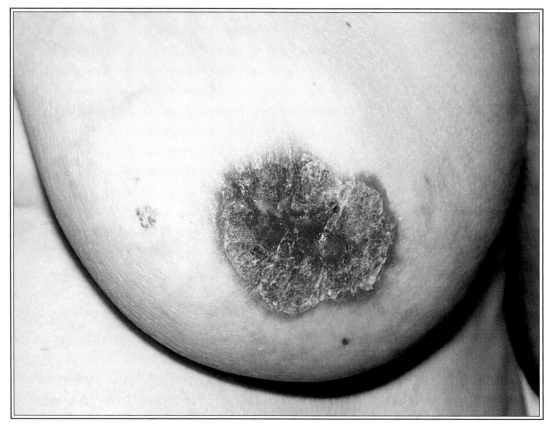

Figure 4

Tether. Skin tether underneath the nipple is easily seen.

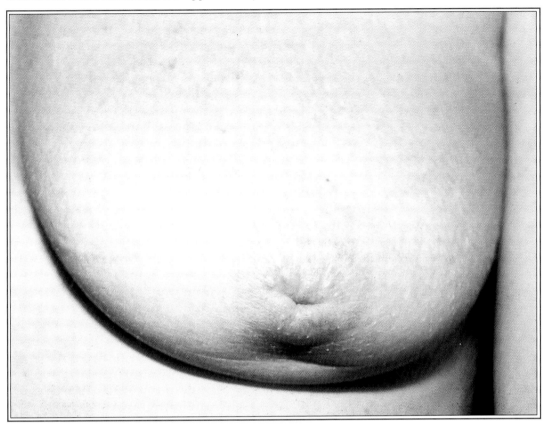

Figure 5

Skin tether may be a much more subtle clinical sign, sometimes seen only when the patient raises her arms above her head.

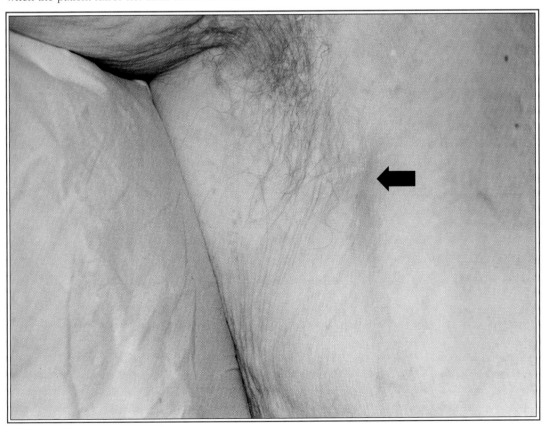

Figure 6

Tether of the nipple. Inpulling of the left nipple is easily seen.

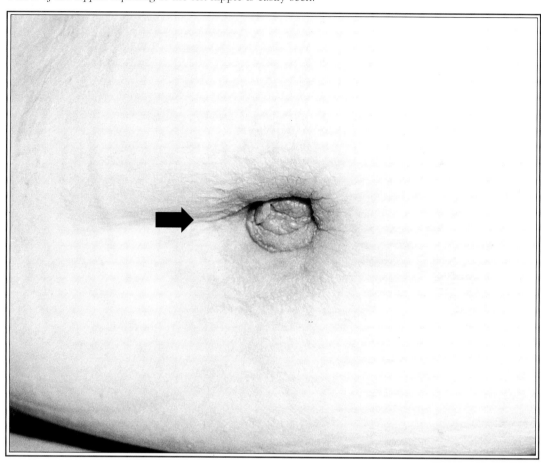

Figure 7

Inspection. The examiner should stand directly in front of the patient who sits on the edge of the examination couch. The breasts are inspected with the arms by the side and then the patient slowly raises her arms and places them behind her head.

Figure 8

Palpation. For palpation, the patient is propped up to about 30 degrees. In this position the breast is easiest to examine. If the patient is lying flat, the skin over the breast becomes more tense and the breast tissue is not as easy to palpate. The patient should be examined first with her arms by her sides, then with her arms placed on her head, and finally sitting up and leaning forward.

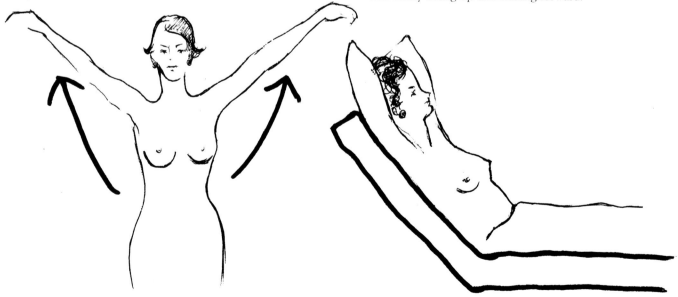

Figure 9

Palpation. Palpation is with the flat of the fingers. The examiner should not press too hard. Some examiners prefer to make a circular movement with the fingers as they feel the breast. Examination should include all quadrants of the breast, the center behind the nipple and the axillary tail.

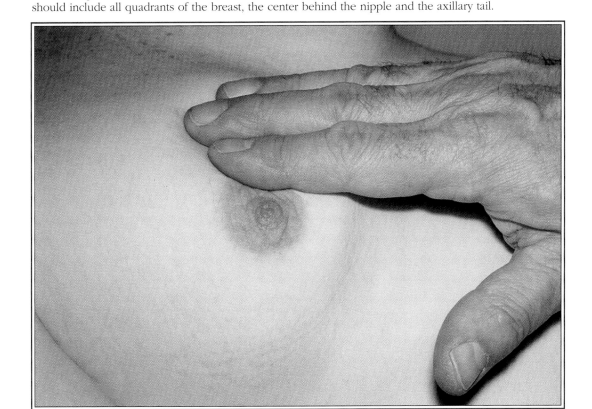

SECTION 2

THE BENIGN LUMP

SECTION 2

CYSTS

Cyst formation is part of the normal process of involution of the breast. Cysts rarely occur before the age of 35, but the breast tissue of the majority of women in their forties will show microscopic cysts, a proportion of which expand to present as clinical lumps. Cysts are easily recognized on ultrasound (Figure 10) and are often detected at mammographic screening as masses in the breast; however, as long as the lesion has all the characteristics of a benign mass, the patient need not be recalled for further assessment (Figure 11). Cysts do not occur in post-menopausal women, although they may persist for some time after the menopause. It should be noted, however, that a woman receiving HRT may not be regarded as post-menopausal from the point of view of the effect on her breast. Cysts have no malignant or premalignant characteristics on histology (Figure 12); they only become important when they form palpable lumps that must be diagnosed. Both diagnosis and treatment is by aspiration; as long as the cyst disappears completely on palpation after aspiration, no further investigation is necessary and the woman can be discharged from the clinic. Any solid lump remaining after aspiration is investigated as described below.

FIBROADENOMAS

Fibroadenomas have a very different age scatter from cysts and are very different in appearance. They occur from the menarche and are most common below the age of 30, although there is a small peak of reappearance in the mid 40s. Fibroadenomas do not occur as new lesions after the menopause; any found at later screening may have been there for several years. They are probably extremely common breast lesions, but as their size distribution is pyramidal, few become detectable lumps.

A fibroadenoma presents commonly as a small, very mobile lump in the breast (breast mouse) that is ovoid in shape and measures 1-2 cm. The cut surface of a fibroadenoma removed at operation is white and bulges freely (Figure 13). Fibroadenomas may be visable on mammography (Figure 14); ultrasound (Figure 15) shows a well defined mass with a homogenous internal echo pattern. Fine needle aspiration (FNA) cytology reveals clumps of benign epithelial cells (Figure 16). Once a fibroadenoma is removed, its characteristics are easily apparent on histology. Cysts, as has been stated are now dealt with by aspiration, but until recently most clinics removed all solid lumps, to ensure they were not malignant. Depending on the clinical feel, imaging and cytological characteristics, the majority of benign lumps are now left in situ in our clinic. This requires very careful investigation and rigorous application of criteria that have been formulated for leaving a benign lump in situ (Table II). The results of applying these criteria are shown in Table III.

Figure 10

Cysts. The differential diagnosis of a non-calcified well-defined mass includes fibroadenoma and a simple benign breast cyst.

Ultrasound is extremely useful in differentiating solid from cystic benign breast lesions. Cysts are demonstrated by ultrasound as well-defined anechoic masses with distal bright up as demonstrated. Neither fibroadenomas nor breast cysts should increase in size after the menopause, unless the patient is receiving hormone replacement therapy.

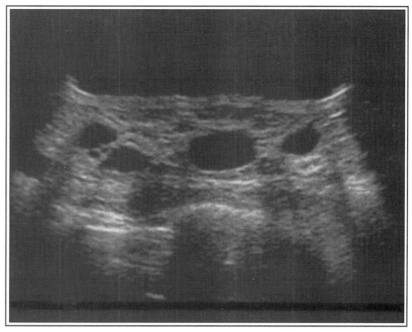

Figure 11

On mammography cysts appear as well defined low density masses. They are often multiple and unlike fibroadenomas are often greater than 3 cm in size. Cysts have a tendency for their long axis orientated towards the nipple.

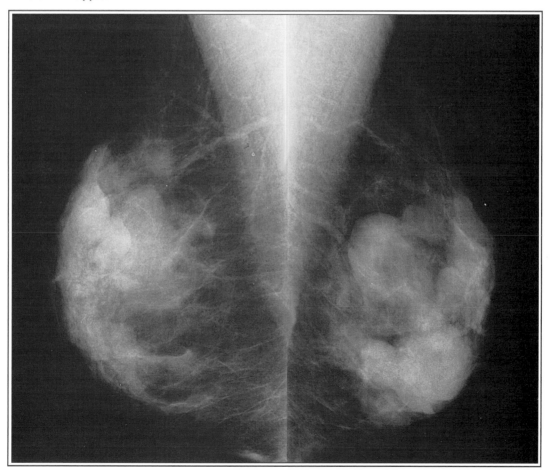

Figure 12

Histological section of a small breast cyst.
The commonest type of breast cyst is lined by a layer of cuboidal or attenuated flattened epithelium as shown in this example. This type of epithelial cell secretes a fluid low in potassium and these cysts tend not to recur after aspiration.

The other common type of breast cyst is lined by a metaplastic apocrine type of epithelium which secretes a fluid rich in potassium. This type is more prone to recurrence after aspiration.

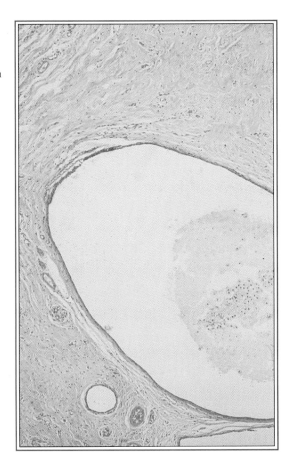

Figure 13

Cut surface of a fibroadenoma. The lesion is seen to be smooth on the outside. The cut surface is white and bulges.

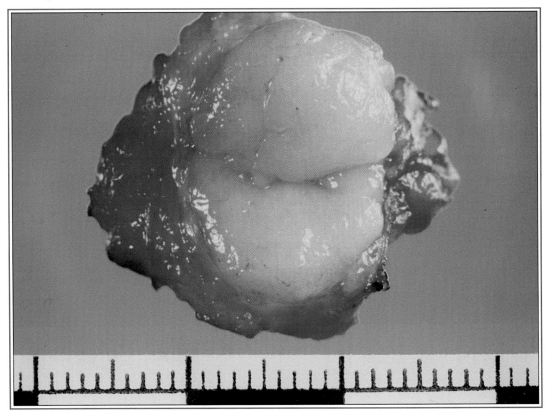

Figure 14

Fibroadenoma. On mammography, fibroadenomas are typically demonstrated as well-defined, rounded and often lobulated masses of variable size. Their density is similar to that of adjacent normal breast tissue.

Calcification is often demonstrated within the fibroadenoma and may be of two types. Most commonly, calcification is associated with hyaline degeneration and is large and dense with a 'popcorn' appearance (as shown here).

Alternatively, calcification situated in entrapped ducts is finer and more granular. Occasionally, the latter type of calcification can be confused with that associated with ductal carcinoma in situ.

Fibroadenomas are often an incidental finding on mammography and may be multiple. In older women, the soft tissue component may not be apparent, leaving only calcifications visible on mammography.

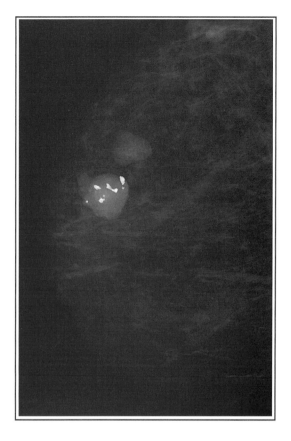

Figure 15

Fibroadenoma. On ultrasound, fibroadenomas are typically well-defined with a lobulated margin and contain an homogeneous reduced internal echo pattern. In younger women (20-30 years), the margins may be less well-defined. Typically, fibroadenomas show either distal acoustic enhancement, particularly in the younger age group, or no distal acoustic changes. However, in older women, fibroadenomas can show distal acoustic shadowing which is usually homogeneous in character. Similarly, calcification within a fibroadenoma may cause localized areas of increased echogenicity and some acoustic shadowing.

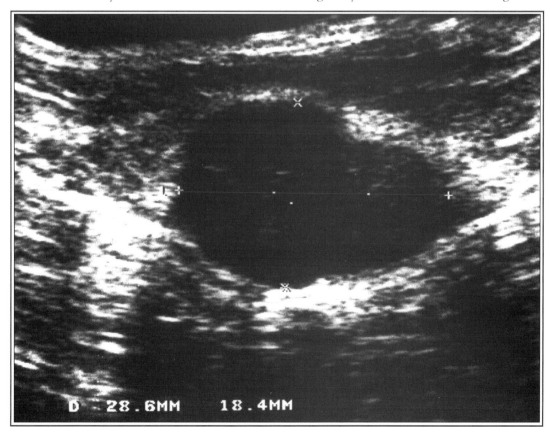

Figure 16

Cytological yield from a fibroadenoma. This is an air-dried preparation stained with a Giemsa stain. The three components of a fibroadenoma can be seen. There are large sheets of tightly cohesive epithelial cells arranged in a regular pattern.

A fragment of stromal tissue of the intralobular type is stained purple.

In addition, there is a dispersed population of so-called bipolar nuclei. These have been stripped from surrounding cytoplasm and although their origin is uncertain, they are likely to be from epithelial, myoepithelial or stromal cells.

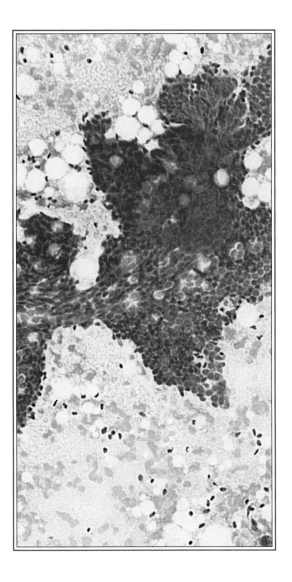

Table II

Criteria by which a palpable solid breast lump may be left in situ. If any one is not satisfied the lump is excised for histological diagnosis. The criteria shown are for women aged 35 and over. For younger women they are less strict. For women under 25, only one fine needle aspirate is taken and excision biopsy would be undertaken only if cytology showed suspicious cells.

CLINICAL	Feel entirely benign - smooth and mobile
IMAGING	Appear benign or no image on mammography
CYTOLOGY	Two FNAs 4-6 weeks apart must both show benign epithelial cells
FOLLOW-UP	At 3 and 6 months, lumps should not have grown significantly

Figure 17

Fibroadenomas. Fibroadenomas are now believed to be localized areas of hyperplasia within the breast, rather than true tumors. They are composed of the tissues present in the normal terminal duct lobular unit (TDLU), that is, epithelial and myoepithelial lined glandular ductal or cleft like spaces surrounded by a loose stromal tissue identical in appearance to intralobular stroma. Fibroadenomas typically have a rounded contour with a pushing margin.

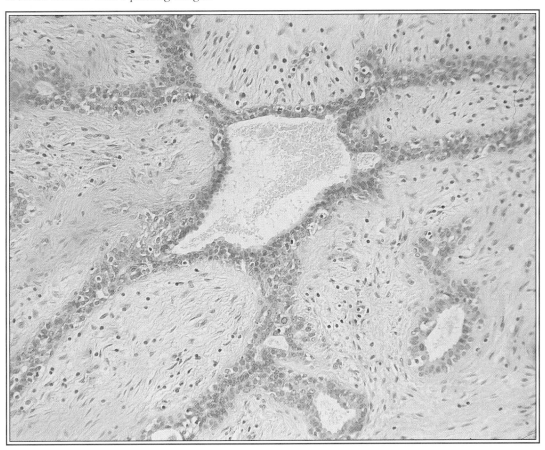

Table III

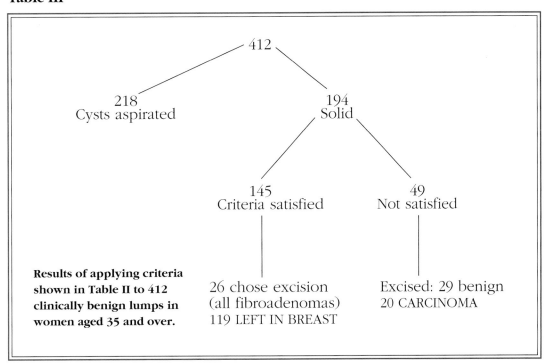

Results of applying criteria shown in Table II to 412 clinically benign lumps in women aged 35 and over.

412

218 Cysts aspirated

194 Solid

145 Criteria satisfied

49 Not satisfied

26 chose excision (all fibroadenomas)
119 LEFT IN BREAST

Excised: 29 benign
20 CARCINOMA

SECTION 3

THE NIPPLE

SECTION 3

THE NIPPLE
Indrawing
Patients are often referred to specialists because of apparent indrawing at the nipple. This is most frequently because the referring practitioner is uncertain of the variations in the appearance of the normal nipple (Figure 18). Normal nipples are frequently indrawn in a line (smile across the nipple), particularly in young women. Alternatively, in old age, one duct at the nipple may become shortened, suggesting tethering of the very center (Figure 19).

Eczema
A true eczematous appearance of the nipple (Figure 20), with excoriation, may indicate Paget's disease and requires a biopsy. This can be undertaken in the clinic using a size 11 scalpel blade held between the fingers. Local anesthetic with adrenaline is put into the nipple and two parallel cuts made around 2 mm apart. The tissue between the cuts is picked up with a small hypodermic needle and cut off. The histological appearance of Paget's disease is characteristic (Figure 21). The appearance of Paget's cells at the nipple, in the absence of a palpable lump, indicates underlying ductal carcinoma in situ, often at the periphery of the breast.

Nipple discharge
Bilateral and often milky discharge from several ducts of the nipple is to be disregarded. This is a physiological upset and does not indicate a pathological lesion. However, discharge from a single duct (Figure 22) indicates that diagnostic tests are appropriate.

Some years ago, we used to carry out the operation of michrodochectomy - removal of the discharging duct-in order to make the diagnosis. In our series, 170 patients with single duct nipple discharges underwent michrodochectomy, but only 12 small carcinomas in situ were found. Most commonly, the discharge was due to duct ectasia (dilatation and thickening of the ducts) (Figure 23) or to small papillomas (Figure 24); neither of these lesions is pre-malignant. Furthermore, the ductal carcinoma in situ was visible on mammography (Figure 25). We have therefore changed our management protocol for single duct nipple discharge; we now carry out careful mammography and only explore the duct if this shows an abnormality.

Duct ectasia/periareolar abscess/mammillary fistula
This title indicates a progression. Ectatic ducts may accumulate static secretion which, if it becomes infected, may lead to an indolent abscess close to the nipple (Figure 26). The abscess may then present acutely and discharge externally, causing a mammillary fistula between the skin and the duct (Figure 27). Alternatively, the lesion may be more indolent and present as an ill-defined lump, somewhat but not acutely tender, beside the nipple. A mammillary fistula is annoying since it gives a continuing discharge. It is treated by placing a probe along its length (Figure 28) which comes out at the nipple. An incision is then made along the length of the probe and the area left open to granulate (Figure 29); acute or chronic periaroelar abscess is treated similarly.

Figure 18

A benign cleft lying horizontally across the nipple.
This feature is commonly seen in the breast clinic.
Patients may be referred for this abnormality, but it
does not indicate underlying pathology.

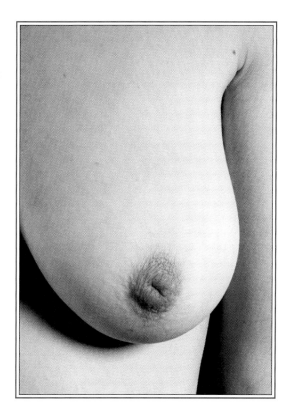

Figure 19

One duct retracted at the center of the nipple. This appearance is often seen in elderly women.

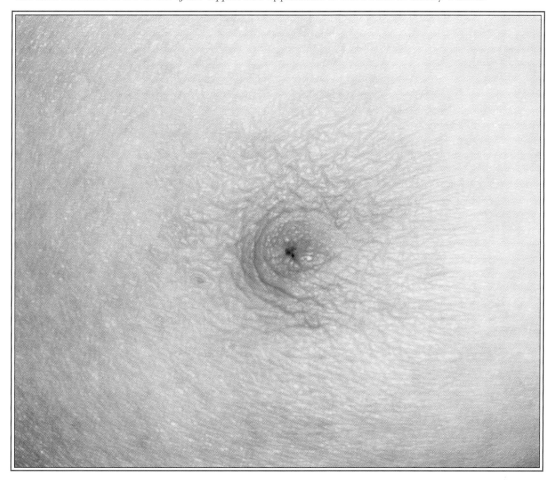

Figure 20

Paget's disease of the nipple. Although there is only a small area of excoriation, biopsy showed this to be Paget's disease of the nipple. Any area of eczematous change of the nipple should be biopsied. Paget's disease of the nipple may heal between episodes of excoriation and a recent history of excoriation is also an indication for biopsy.

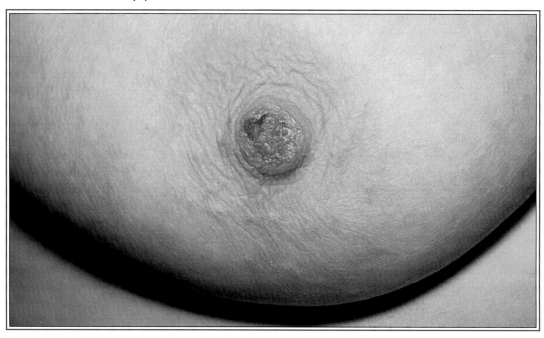

Figure 21

Histological section of the epidermis of the nipple in a case of Paget's disease. The stratified squamous epithelium shows infiltration by a population of large pleomorphic cells with a high nuclear cytoplasmic ratio. There is usually direct continuity between the area of the nipple involved and underlying nipple ducts containing DCIS.

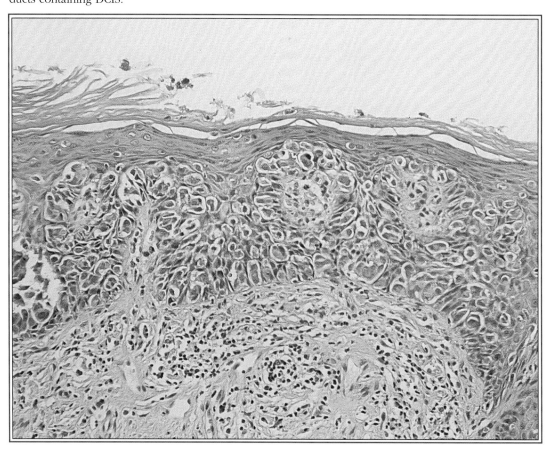

Figure 22

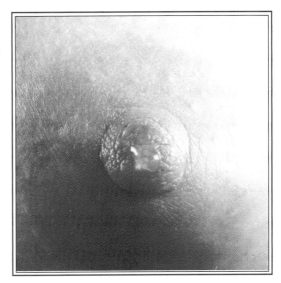

Single duct nipple discharge. Whether the discharge is clear or contains blood is not as useful a diagnostic sign as is often quoted. It is more important to discover whether a palpable or mammographic abnormality is present.

If cytology of the discharge is carried out and obvious cancer cells are found, clearly an underlying breast cancer is indicated. However, suspicious cells found in nipple discharge are often merely degenerate duct cells.

Figure 23

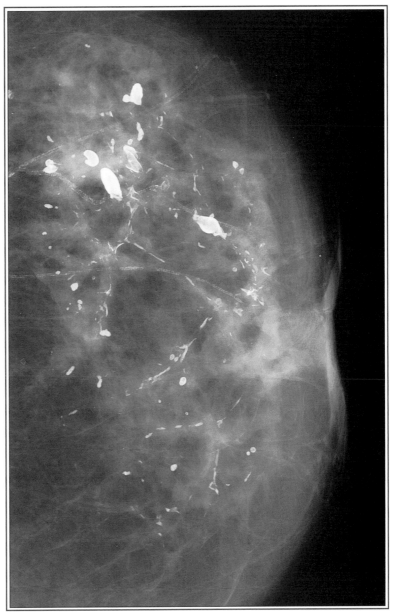

Duct ectasia.
On mammography, duct ectasia is commonly manifested as rod-like dense calcifications in a ductal distribution (broken needle appearance).

Calcification can also be shown in the periductal tissues where it may have a central lucency.
The calcifications of duct ectasia can occasionally be confused with those of ductal carcinoma in situ. However, the latter are normally finer, granular and more pleomorphic.

Calcifications due to fat necrosis are often seen in association with those of duct ectasia (as in this case).

Figure 24

Histological section of a duct papilloma. Papillomas have a fronded configuration and are lined by the normal bilayer of cells found in the breast, that is an epithelial and a myoepithelial layer. They are supported by a vascular stroma. In some papillomas, epithelial hyperplasia may occur and is recognized by an increase in the number of epithelial cells above the single myoepithelial layer (not present in this illustration).

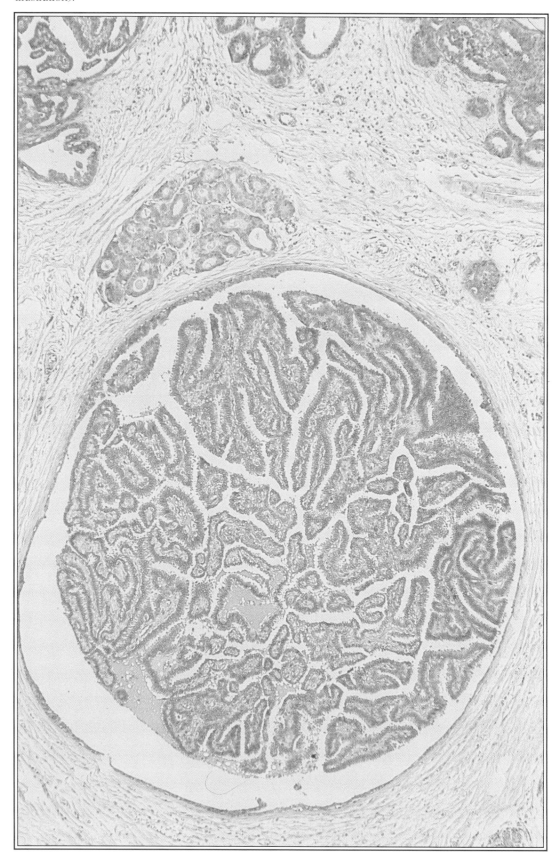

Figure 25

Ductal carcinoma in situ. This mammogram was taken because the patient was complaining of single duct nipple discharge and no lump was palpable. The most common manifestation of ductal carcinoma in situ (DCIS) on mammography is microcalcifications, with or without an associated soft tissue density. The classical appearance is of irregular elongated rod or Y-shaped calcifications which occur in a ductal distribution. There is often a wide variation in size, density and shape of these calcifications.

The calcifications are normally in an irregularly shaped cluster. This appearance is most often seen in comedo type DCIS. The cribriform, small-cell type of DCIS can manifest as small, granular microcalcifications which can be easily confused with these associated with microcystic change or sclerosing adenosis. Small-cell DCIS is more often occult than the comedo type. It is also more likely to manifest as a soft-tissue mass without calcification.

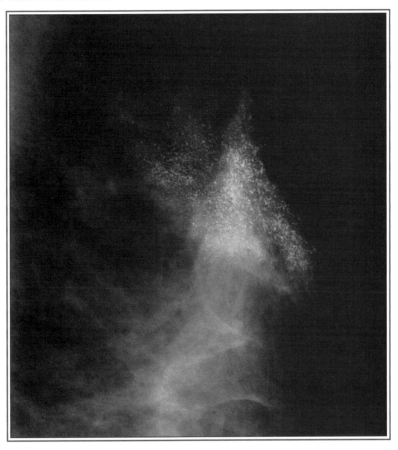

Figure 26

Peri-areolar abscess. An area of inflammation around the edge of the areola indicates a peri-areolar abscess arising from infection within duct ectasia.

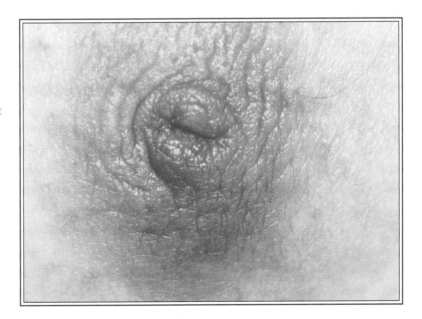

Figure 27

Mammillary fistula.
This appearance is
characteristic.

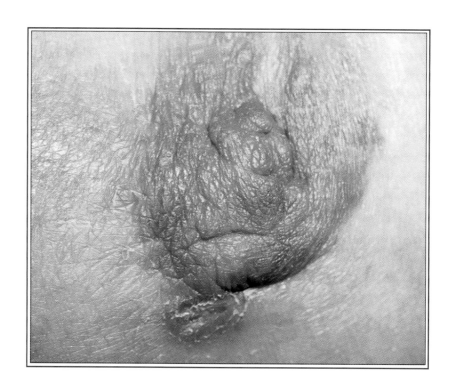

Figure 28

The treatment of mammillary fistula. A probe is placed into the fistula and appears through the nipple.

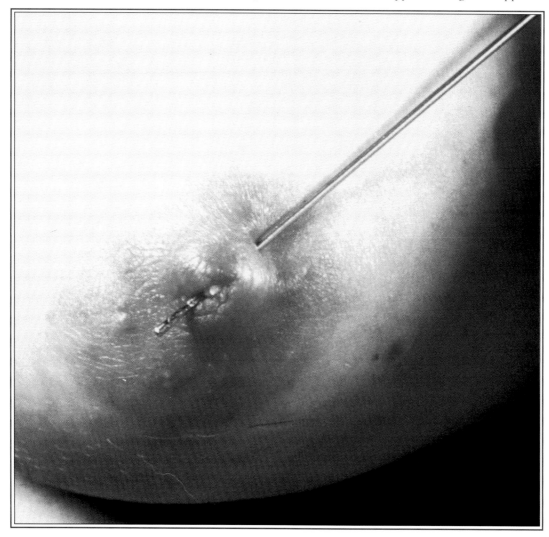

Figure 29

Treatment of a mammillary fistula. A cut is made along the probe and the wound left to granulate.

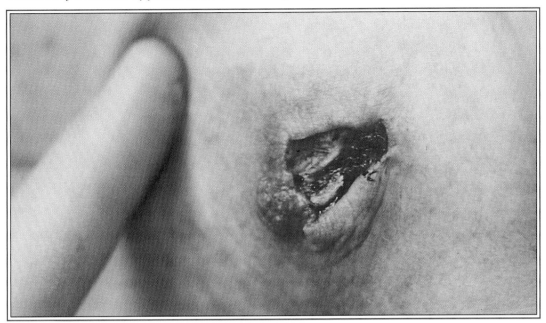

SECTION 4

PRIMARY BREAST CANCER

SECTION 4

PRIMARY BREAST CANCER

Primary breast cancer (Figures 30 and 31) usually presents as a solid lump in the breast. The other presentations-skin and nipple tether, nipple discharge and nipple eczema-have already been mentioned. Since the advent of screening, a number of breast cancers which have no clinical signs have been discovered and will be referred to later. Breast cancers may have a number of appearances on mammography (Figures 32-34) and on ultrasound (Figure 35).

Diagnosis is made by needle histology of the lump (Figures 36 & 37) or by fine needle aspiration (Figure 38). The determination of whether a lump is benign or malignant should ideally be made at the very first attendance. If the diagnosis is cancer, once the surgeon has explained it to the patient, she should be seen by a breast care nurse (Figure 39) who is able to talk with her at length and explain the treatment options available. In this way, the patient is able to participate in choosing her treatment. Even if the recommended treatment is straightforward and no other options are appropriate, a breast nurse can still help explain to the patient what will happen to her.

Treatment options have become widely available for most women, particularly over the last 10 years. In the first 60 years of this century breast cancer was uniformly treated by radical mastectomy (sometimes modified radical) followed by irradiation of the chest wall. This gave rise to many problems, an example of which is shown in Figure 40. In addition, the axilla was completely dissected up to the first rib and then radiotherapy given to the axilla, frequently giving rise to lymphoedema of the arm (Figure 41) and to other problems. Indeed, it could be argued that during this time the mode of treatment did more harm than good.

As a result of the clinical trials of the 1960s, simple (total) mastectomy became widely used in the 1970s and prophylactic treatment of the axilla is often now omitted (see below). Simple mastectomy produces a better cosmetic result than radical mastectomy (Figure 42), but of course there is still no breast. Possible methods of reconstructing the breast include subcutaneous mastectomy followed by insertion of a silicone implant (Figure 43), and more extensive reconstruction, involving musculo-cutaneous flaps, which are necessary when a total mastectomy has been undertaken.

Surgery with breast conservation was originally described by Geoffrey Keynes, a surgeon at St. Bartholomew's Hospital, London, in the 1930s. However, the technique did not begin to have wide appeal until Calle and his colleagues, at the Institut Curie in Paris, began to reintroduce it in the 1960s. In the 1980s, treatment of breast cancer with breast conservation became perhaps the most common method of treating operable primary breast cancer, certainly in women under the age of 70, and a good cosmetic result may be achieved. Figure 44 shows the result in a woman treated in Nottingham by excision of a tumor in the left breast with margins apparently free of tumor histologically, followed by intact breast irradiation. This is by no means an unusual example of the cosmetic results achieved at our center.

However, because of the danger of recurrences in the treated breast, a number of precautions have to be observed. It is unwise to use this technique on larger tumors (we restrict it to tumors of 3 cm or less). At operation, the intention is to achieve apparently clear margins on histology, while preserving a reasonable cosmetic appearance and therefore not excising too much tissue. The surgeon aims to take 1-1$^{1}/_{2}$ cm around the palpable edge of the tumor.

A specimen X-ray is taken to ensure that the margins appear clear around the tumor (Figure 45). The specimen is carefully orientated and the exterior is inked so that the pathologist can see the edge at histology and examine the margins for the presence of tumor. If tumor is found at the margin of excision, re-excision of that edge is undertaken.

The alternative operative technique is to carry out quadrantectomy (segmentectomy), or removal of up to a quarter of the breast. Although when used in small tumors (no bigger than 2 cm) and followed by radiotherapy this gives a low rate of recurrence in the treated breast, the cosmetic result is often poor and plastic surgery may be required (Figure 46). Because breast conservation is carried out in preference to mastectomy purely for cosmetic reasons, there seems little point in doing it unless the final appearence is good. For that reason, we prefer the wide local excision technique described.

To avoid local recurrence in the treated breast after wide local excision, and particularly to avoid local recurrence of a very unpleasant kind, where the whole breast is suddenly found to be infiltrated with tumor (Figure 47), a number of criteria have to be observed. The initial size of the tumor and the completeness of excision on histology have been referred to already. In addition, the specimen is examined for the presence of vascular invasion, that is a tumor within small blood vessels or lymphatics (Figure 48), in or around the primary tumor. In some units, the presence of extensive ductal carcinoma in situ within and around the primary invasive tumor is considered to indicate that local recurrence is likely. If vascular invasion is present and the woman is young, particularly 40 or less but even up to 50, she is at much greater danger of recurrence in the treated breast, even after radiotherapy, and the tumor is better treated with mastectomy. Following breast conservation, the patient must be followed up with regular clinical examinations and with mammography of the treated breast biennially, certainly for 10 years (Figures 49 & 50). The patient should also be warned at the outset that any suspicious areas found clinically or mammographically during follow-up are likely to be examined by FNA cytology. It is important that any recurrence be treated early, in order that the tumor should not grow to become larger than the original primary tumor; if this occurs (and only then) the chances of survival appear to be worsened by local recurrence.

PROGNOSIS OF A PRIMARY BREAST CANCER
Parameters to be measured
The lymph nodes should be sampled whether breast cancer is treated by mastectomy

or by breast conservation. Most units sample only axillary lymph nodes, but some also sample the internal mammary nodes in inner-half tumors. Sampling determines lymph node involvement, a time-dependent prognostic factor. Careful measurement of the other time-dependent factor, size of tumor at histology, adds somewhat to prognostic accuracy. However, accurate prognosis also requires information about the natural aggressiveness of the tumor, which is best obtained from histological grading (Figures 51 & 52). Information about whether hormonal treatment is likely to be useful in the later management of the patient can be obtained by staining the tumor for the presence of estrogen receptor (Figure 53). Once all this information has been gathered, the prognosis for the individual may be estimated.

A simple way to do this is to combine lymph node stage and tumor grade and size into the Nottingham Prognostic Index (Figure 54). A forecast can then be made of whether the patient has a very good life expectancy 15-20 years after treatment, a very poor life expectancy, or a breast cancer that gives good survival chances at five years, but from which it is likely that she will succumb in the end.

Selection for adjuvant systemic therapy

The prognosis can be used to help determine which, if any, adjuvant systemic treatment to use in order to combat distant metastases. If, as is the case in the excellent and good prognostic groups (Figure 54), it is unlikely that distant metastases are present, cytotoxic treatment is certainly not indicated nor, arguably, is hormonal treatment.

There is, in the excellent prognostic group, only a 10% chance of dying from breast cancer by 15 years. On the other hand, in the poor prognostic group, it is likely that the tumor will be aggressive and estrogen receptor negative on staining, with the patient standing a high chance of dying of breast cancer within the first 5-7 years. Cytotoxic therapy is indicated in this group if the patient is fit enough to face it. The appropriate method of adjuvant systemic treatment in the moderate group is debatable, but certainly the use of hormonal therapy should be advised when the tumor is estrogen receptor positive.

Figure 30

Cross section of an invasive adenocarcinoma of the breast. The configuration is typical for many breast tumors, with spicules radiating out from a central mass lesion. This appearance gives cancer its name - 'the crab'.

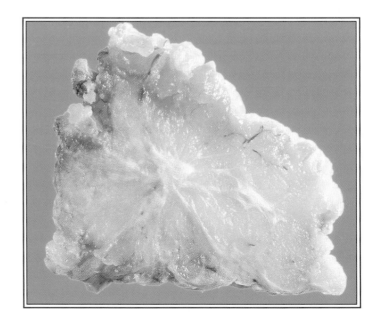

Figure 31

A lump and tether seen close to the nipple. Clinically, this could be nothing other than a breast cancer.

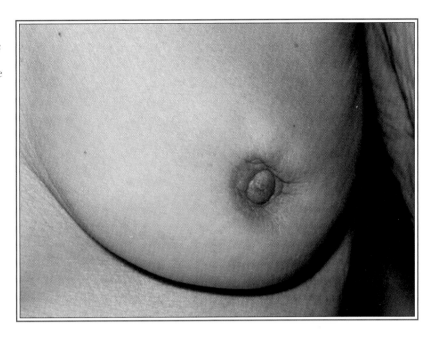

Figure 32

Primary breast cancer. The large variety of appearances of breast carcinoma on mammography can be simply classified into five sub-groups:

♦ *mass* ♦ *spiculate mass* ♦ *architectural distortion or stellate lesions* ♦ *asymmetry* ♦ *calcification*

This mammogram shows the classical appearance of a carcinoma on mammography - a spiculate mass. There is a definable central mass with irregular margins and distortion of the surrounding tissue. Spicules and tentacles seen around the central mass represent a desmoplastic reaction associated with the tumor. Microcalcifications within and around the tumor mass are seen in approximately one third of cases and are typical of associated ductal carcinoma in situ. A spiculate mass with associated calcifications has a 95% chance of being malignant. The differential diagnosis includes localized sclerosing adenosis, scar from previous surgery, radial scar/complex sclerosing lesion and localized fat necrosis.

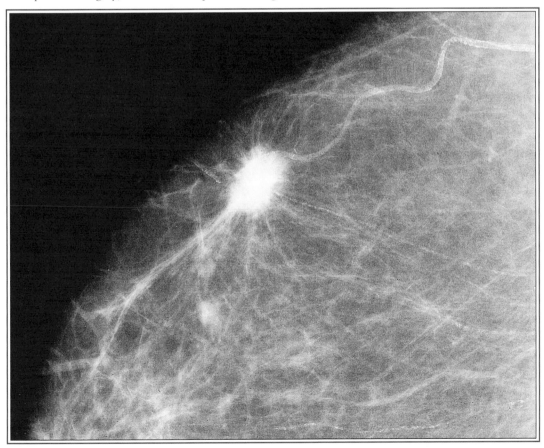

Figure 33

Primary breast carcinoma. Mammography on this page shows two carcinomas. Firstly there is an obvious, slightly ill-defined soft tissue mass in the left breast with associated skin thickening. In addition, within the right breast there is an area of distortion and increased density in the lateral part of the breast disk. Parenchymal distortion is one of the most important features of early breast carcinoma.

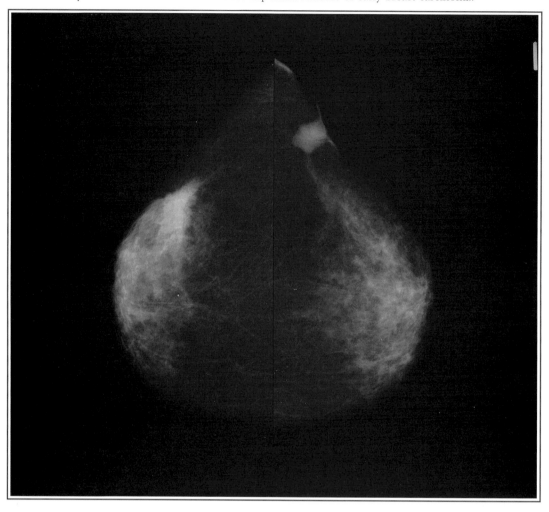

Figure 34

Primary breast carcinoma. This mammogram demonstrates a dense parenchymal pattern which can make detection of breast cancer more difficult. Two particularly helpful signs in dense breasts are parenchymal distortion (shown here centrally within the right breast) and abnormal microcalcifications.

Cancers producing parenchymal distortion without any central mass (as in this case) are often of the tubular type and usually carry an excellent prognosis. The differential diagnosis of such an appearance is a radial scar/complex sclerosing lesion.

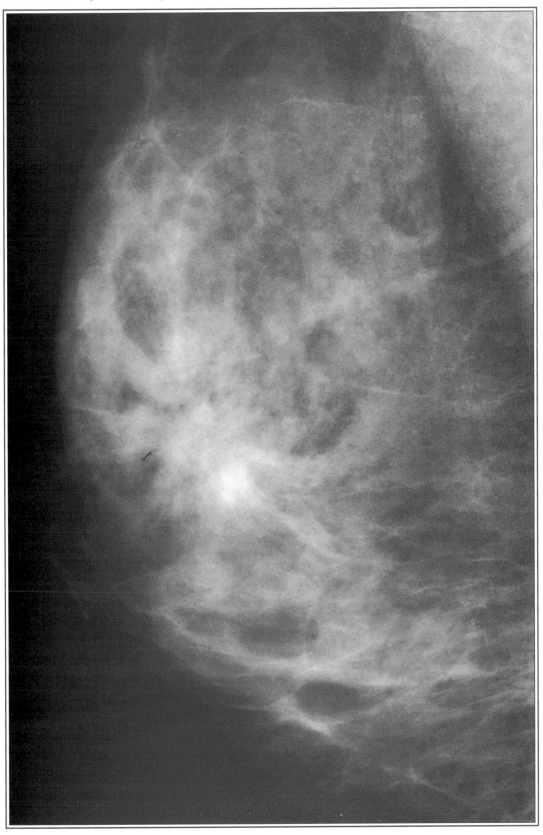

Figure 35

Ultrasound of breast carcinoma. Carcinoma of the breast typically appears as shown, an irregular mass of reduced and mixed echogenicity with distal acoustic shadowing - in contrast to the typical appearance of a benign cyst or fibroadenoma. Additional features may include a 'halo' of increased echogenicity and distortion of the surrounding normal breast parenchyma. Ultrasound is very useful for confirming the diagnosis of malignancy, but cannot be used to definitively differentiate benign from malignant solid lesions in the breast.

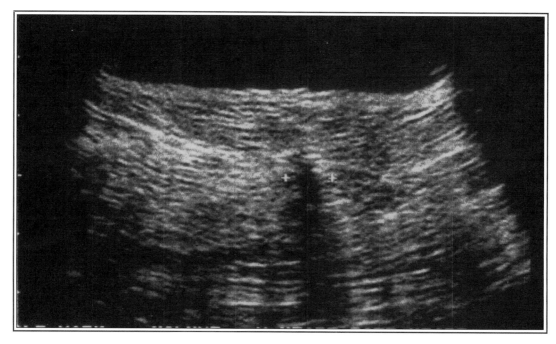

Figure 36

Biopsy needle histology. The skin over the lesion and the lesion itself are locally anesthetized. A small cut is made in the skin with a pointed no.11 scalpel blade and then a Trucut needle is inserted up as far as the lump. The central core needle then cuts into the lump and a sheath is pushed forward over it.

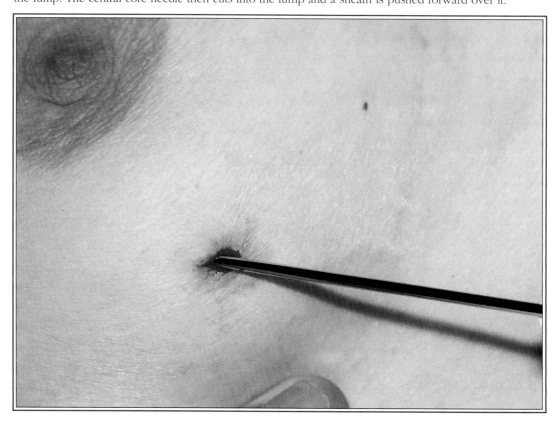

Figure 37

A piece of tumor in the slot of the Trucut needle. This is suitable for histological examination.

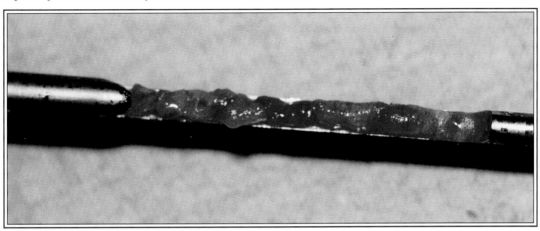

Figure 38

A fine needle aspiration cytology sample from a breast carcinoma (air dried Giemsa stain). One of the properties of normal epithelial cells is strong cell-to-cell cohesion which on FNA cytology sampling leads to the arrangement of benign cells as large tightly cohesive groups (see Figure 16).

In carcinoma cell populations this cell-to-cell cohesion is reduced. For this reason it is often possible to get a high cell yield from an aspirate sample and the cells obtained when smeared are dispersed across the slide as shown. Normal cells have a regular appearance, in contrast to carcinoma cells which show an increase in cell size, high nuclear:cytoplasmic ratio and pleomorphism of nuclear morphology.

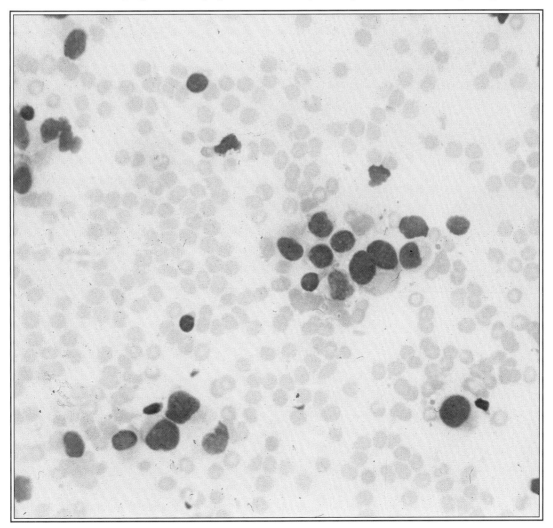

Figure 39

Breast care nurse. Women given the diagnosis of breast cancer by the surgeon should have an opportunity to talk with the breast care nurse about their disease and the options for treatment. The patient is then able to participate in the choice of treatment.

Post-operatively, the breast care nurse should be seen by the patient as a friend who is able to 'translate' medical advice. She should be responsible for recognizing depression and anxiety and for onward referral to a psychiatrist or conducting counselling as necessary.

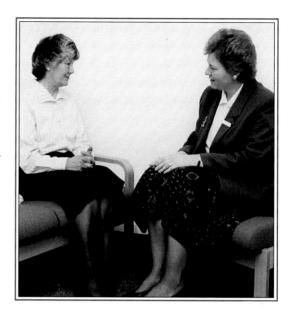

Figure 40

Radical mastectomy. An example of the possible outcome when radical mastectomy followed by irradiation of the chest wall and axilla was the standard treatment for breast cancer. Radiation necrosis of the skin of the chest wall is seen. Fractures of the ribs and fibrosis of the lung also occurred.

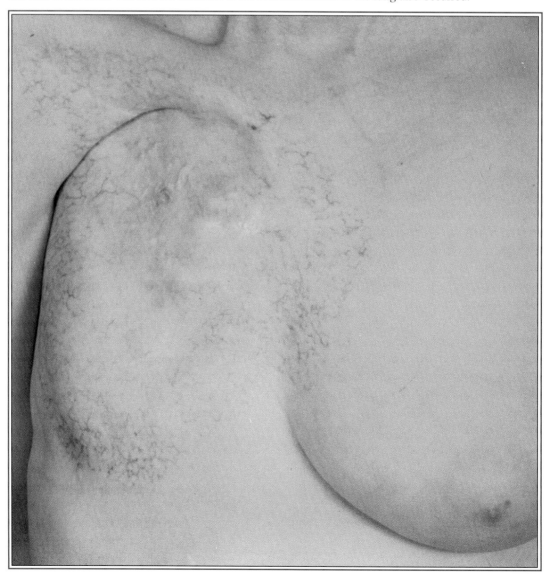

Figure 41

Lymphoedema of the arm. This was common when complete axillary dissection, followed by radiation, was the standard treatment for breast cancer.

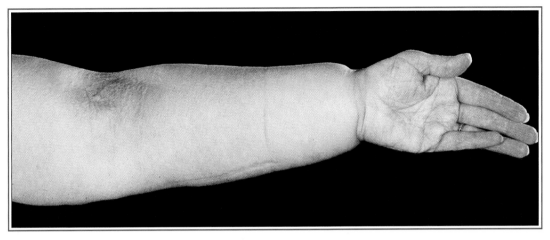

Figure 42

Simple (total) mastectomy. This became the standard treatment for breast cancer in the 1960s following a number of clinical trials which demonstrated that the survival outcome was no better in patients who had undergone radical mastectomy or mastectomy with irradiation than in those who underwent simple mastectomy alone.

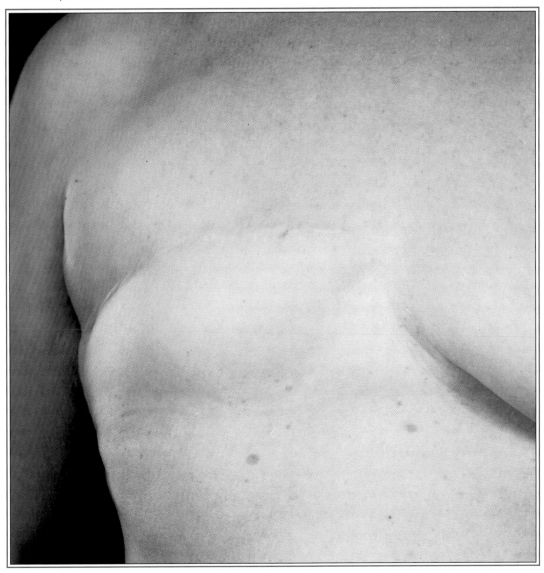

Figure 43

Subcutaneous mastectomy for breast cancer followed by a silicone implant. This has been carried out on the left side; the left nipple faces a little outwards because of the shape of the prosthesis used.

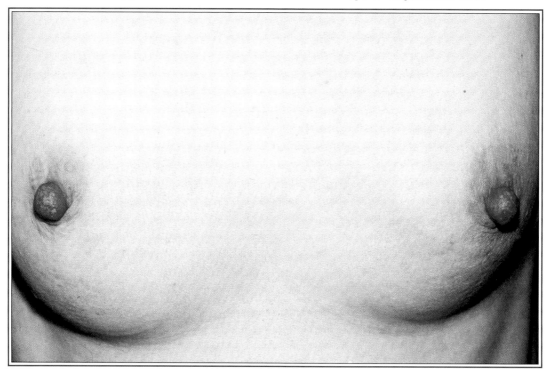

Figure 44

Breast conservation. A typical example of a woman who has undergone breast conservation by wide local excision of the tumor to clear histological margins followed by intact breast irradiation. At operation, the surgeon aims for a palpable margin of around 1-1.5 cm. If the margin is less than 0.5 cm on histology, re-excision is undertaken.

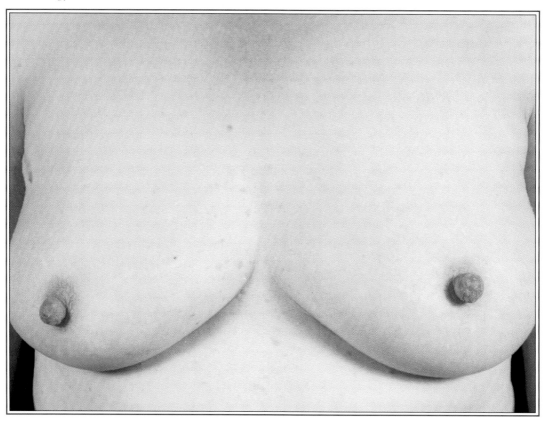

Figure 45

Specimen X-ray of a breast cancer excised by wide local excision. The surgeon checks that the margins are not too close. On this occasion, re-excision of the lower lateral margin (this tumor is on the left side) might have been carried out at the original operation. The ultimate check, however, is by the pathologist.

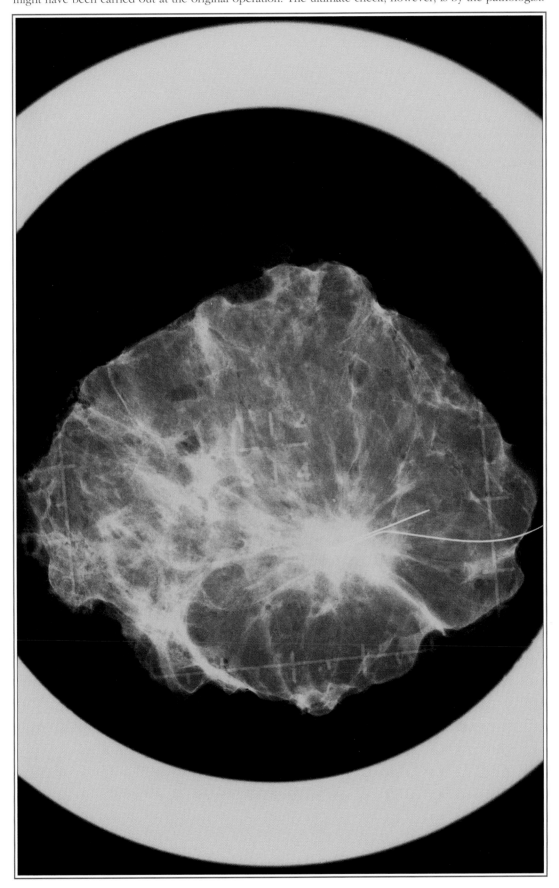

Figure 46

The cosmetic result of quadrantectomy. A large part of the breast is removed in this operation, giving rise to a cosmetic defect.

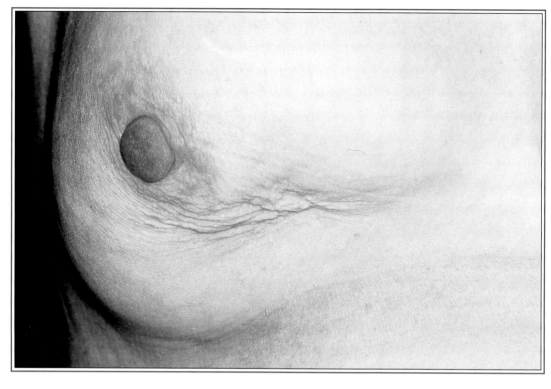

Figure 47

Aggressive, uncontrollable type of local recurrence that occasionally follows treatment for breast cancer with breast conservation. Now that new selection criteria have been established for suitability for treatment with breast conservation, this type of recurrence has been completely abolished in our center.

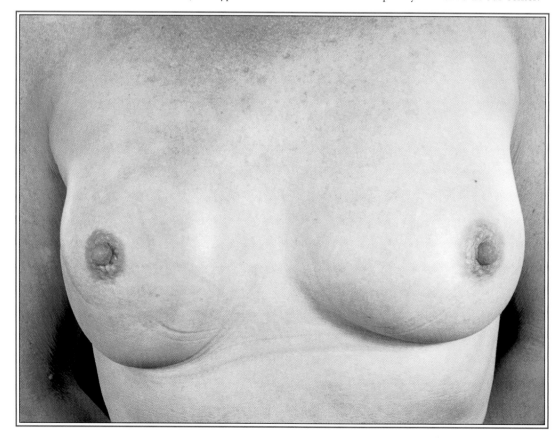

Figure 48

Histological section from tissue adjacent to an invasive adenocarcinoma of the breast. The slide shows a small vessel, most probably a lymphatic channel, containing a focus of tumor cells. The vascular space can be identified by the presence of an endothelial cell lining. The presence of tumor foci within the blood vessels is a poor prognostic feature and associated with the presence of lymph node and distant metastatic disease. In patients treated with conservation therapy, the presence of vascular invasion is associated with a high risk of subsequent local recurrence. There is also an increased risk of recurrence in skin flaps in patients treated by mastectomy.

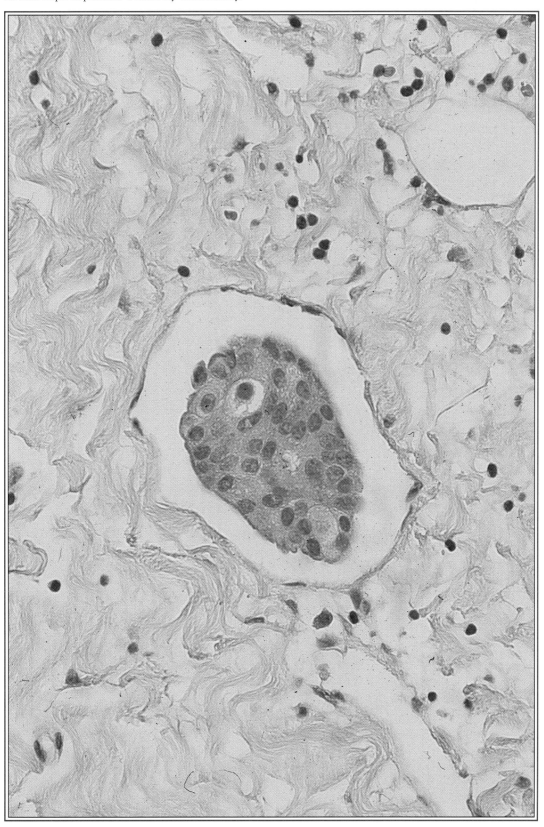

Figure 49 & 50 *Imaging of local recurrence in the conserved breast.*

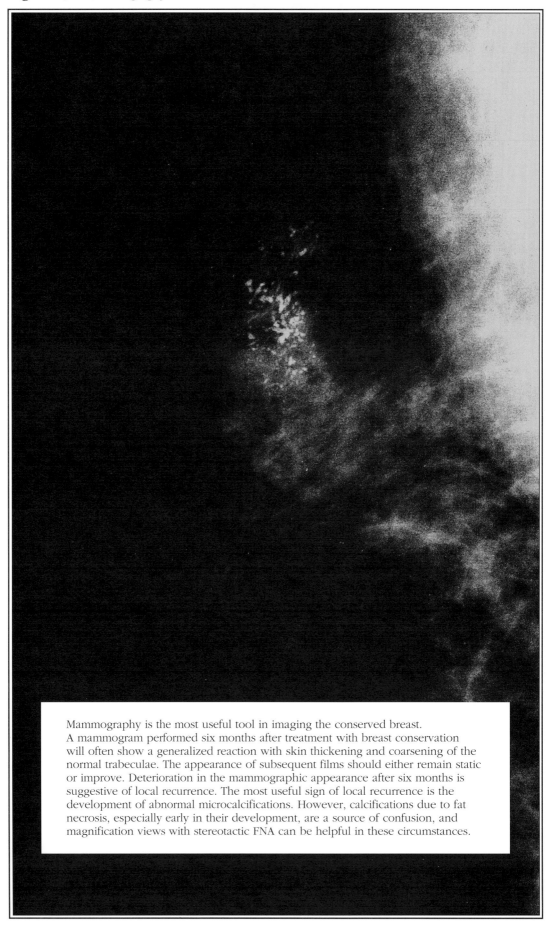

Mammography is the most useful tool in imaging the conserved breast.
A mammogram performed six months after treatment with breast conservation
will often show a generalized reaction with skin thickening and coarsening of the
normal trabeculae. The appearance of subsequent films should either remain static
or improve. Deterioration in the mammographic appearance after six months is
suggestive of local recurrence. The most useful sign of local recurrence is the
development of abnormal microcalcifications. However, calcifications due to fat
necrosis, especially early in their development, are a source of confusion, and
magnification views with stereotactic FNA can be helpful in these circumstances.

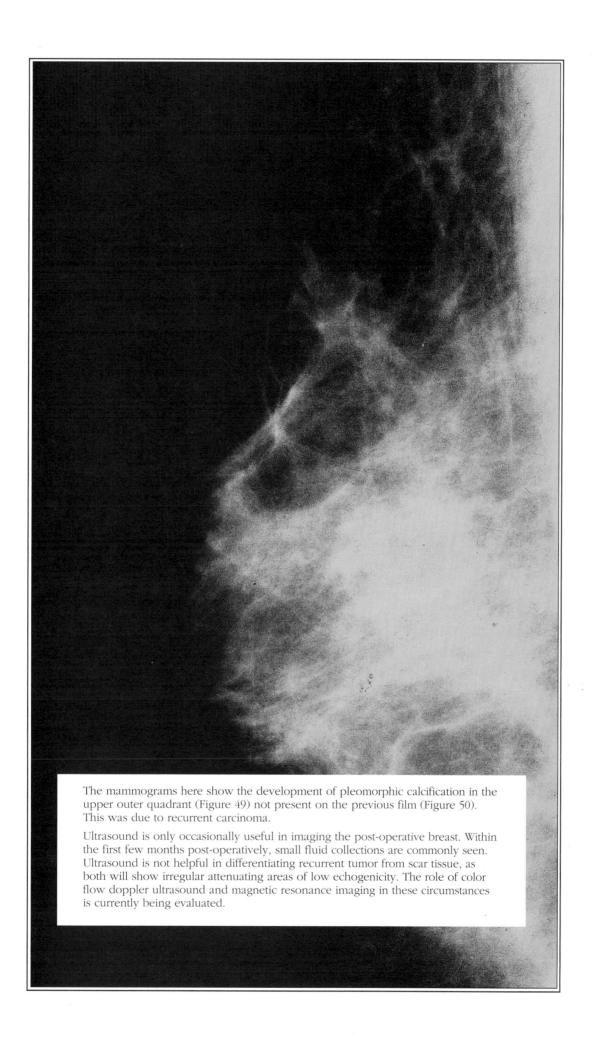

The mammograms here show the development of pleomorphic calcification in the upper outer quadrant (Figure 49) not present on the previous film (Figure 50). This was due to recurrent carcinoma.

Ultrasound is only occasionally useful in imaging the post-operative breast. Within the first few months post-operatively, small fluid collections are commonly seen. Ultrasound is not helpful in differentiating recurrent tumor from scar tissue, as both will show irregular attenuating areas of low echogenicity. The role of color flow doppler ultrasound and magnetic resonance imaging in these circumstances is currently being evaluated.

Figure 51

Histological section of a well-differentiated invasive adenocarcinoma of the breast. Grading or differentiation of breast carcinomas relies on recognition of three features: the formation of glandular or tubular structures, the degree of nuclear pleomorphism, and the frequency of mitotic figures, which are used to assess how closely a tumor cell population resembles the normal terminal duct lobular unit structure of a breast.

In this example, the tumor cells are relatively small and regular in appearance. There are no mitotic figures visible in this field and the tumor cells are forming recognizable glandular structures in places. These characteristics are favorable, indicating a high level of differentiation (grade1).

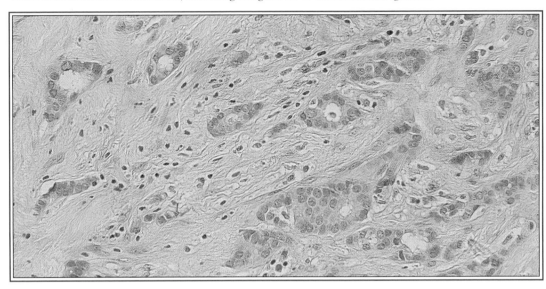

Figure 52

Histological section of a poorly differentiated invasive adenocarcinoma of the breast. In contrast to Figure 51, this tumor is composed of large highly pleomorphic cells, obvious mitotic figures are present within the field and there is no evidence of glandular lumen formation. This tumor would therefore accrue poor scores for the three grade components and have an overall classification of poor differentiation (grade 3).

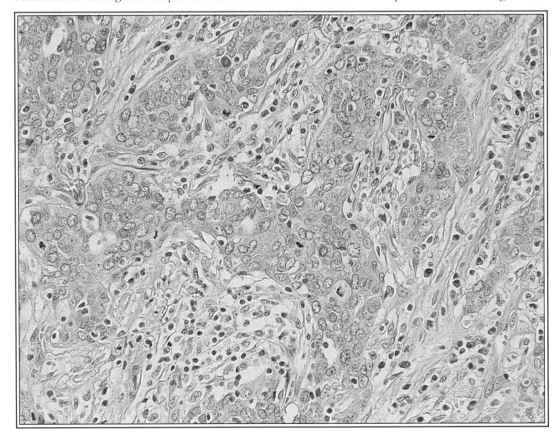

Figure 53

Estrogen receptor immunocytochemical assay (ERICA). This tissue section of an invasive adenocarcinoma of the breast has been stained by an immunocytochemical method using an antibody to the human estrogen receptor located within the nucleus. The method identifies antibody localization with a brown pigment; in this case virtually all the invasive tumor cell nuclei show positive reactivity (brown staining), indicating a high level of expression of estrogen receptor. This tumor would be classified as estrogen receptor positive and would have a high probability of response to hormone therapy.

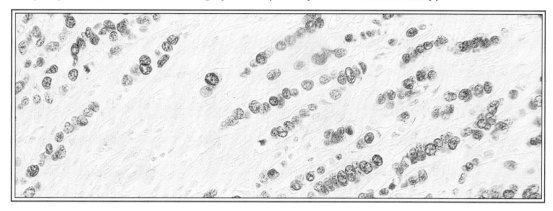

Figure 54

The Nottingham Prognostic Index. The Nottingham Prognostic Index is a combination of tumor size, stage (the presence and level of histological node involvement) and tumor histological grade. This gives excellent prognostic discrimination. For example, it may be seen from this graph that patients placed into the excellent prognostic group (EPG) (around 10% of patients in the symptomatically-presenting population and around 30% of patients in the screened population) have a survival close to that of the age-matched controls. Patients in the moderate prognostic groups (MPG) have approximately a 5-year survival of more than 70% but their survival at 15 years is approximaely 30%. Patients in the poor prognostic group (PPG) have a very poor outlook. These predictions of survival in an individual are relevant to the choice of systemic adjuvant therapies.

The Nottingham Index is the only prospectively validated integrated prognostic index so far published. To get an index value, the index *Grade* is measured by the pathologist by Elston's method which scores mitosis, pleomorphism and tubule formation and from these compiles an overall grade, from I (well differentiated) - III (poor); lymph nodes are sampled *stage* is then measured 1-3 - from no nodes involved (scores 1) to high nodes or both axillary and internal mammary chains involved (3); the tumor *size* on histology is added (cm x 0.2). An index of ≤ 2.4 places a patient in the excellent prognostic group; 2.41-3.4 good; 3.41-5.4 moderate and 5.41+ poor (see survival curves in Figure 54).

Figure 72 shows the percentage of all patients aged 70 or less, with operable breast cancer, falling into each prognostic group. Figure 71 demonstrates the improved prognoses in tumors detected at screening.

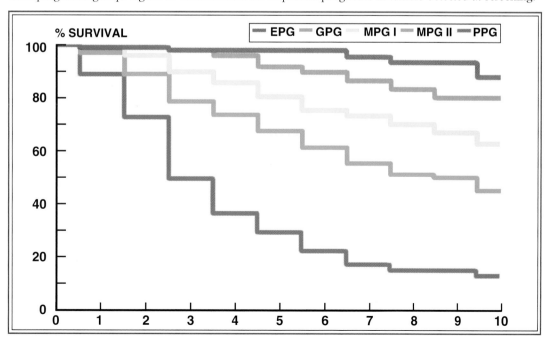

SECTION 5

BREAST CANCER SCREENING

SECTION 5

BREAST CANCER SCREENING

The ability of breast cancer screening to save a number of women from dying of breast cancer has been clearly demonstrated in several randomized trials including the New York Health Insurance Plan (HIP) trial and the Swedish Randomized Trials. The result from one of these was that within a recognized population of randomized controls, 217 deaths would have been expected; in fact, only 160 were observed in the study group (invited for screening). That is to say, of 217 women expected to die of breast cancer, 57 had not done so by nine years. The effect is even greater if only post-menopausal women are taken into account. The significance of the statistics is stronger when the results from all four Swedish screening centers, which carried out randomized trials, are combined.

All trials in women over the age of 50 show an advantage in terms of lower mortality from breast cancer in the populations of women invited for screening. The effect in women under the age of 50 is much less pronounced and does not reach statistical significance. This is generally attributed to the denser mammogram found in pre-menopausal women. As a result of these trials, breast cancer screening has been implemented in the United Kingdom for all women between the ages of 50 and 64. Other countries, including the Netherlands, Italy, Australia, New Zealand and Sweden are currently introducing national screening programs. In the UK, women are invited every three years for screening by mammography only. On the first attendance, two views (craniocaudal and medio-lateral oblique) are performed, but on subsequent attendances the medio-lateral oblique view only is required. Women found to have an abnormality on the mammogram, and those few cases noted by the radiographer to have a clinical abnormality (although there is no formal clinical examination of the breast) are called back for assessment (Figure 55).

At assessment, the following personnel, specially trained in different aspects of breast disease diagnosis should be present: a radiographer, a radiologist and a surgeon, with the opinion of a pathologist for cytology available and a breast care nurse to talk to women who have breast cancer diagnosed or who are worried by the investigation process. There must be facilities for further mammographic views, ultrasound and image-guided fine needle aspirations for cytology or needle biopsy histology of impalpable lesions. Lesions particularly found at breast cancer screening include ductal carcinoma in situ (Figures 56 & 57) and small, well-differentiated invasive carcinomas often of special types (Figures 58 & 59) which have a survival outlook akin to ductal carcinoma in situ.

Ultrasound is used to aid diagnostic needling of impalpable lesions and implantation of wires to guide operative biopsy. Alternatively, a stereotactic device may be added to the mammogram machine (Figure 60) to enable the radiologist to place a needle or a localization wire accurately within the lesion (Figures 61 & 62).

Cytology may show benign cells or give the diagnosis of cancer, enabling the surgeon to proceed to a therapeutic operation (mastectomy or wide excision of the cancer). Benign cytology may provide further reassurance that a lesion thought by the radiologist to have a low chance of being malignant is, in fact, benign. However, certain lesions (Figure 63) judged on imaging to be suspicious, require excision or incision operative biopsy even if the cells aspirated are benign epithelial cells. Stellate lesions of this kind may be tubular carcinomas, or they may be simple benign radial scars (Figure 64) and no further imaging can help in differentiation. Even if benign cells are aspirated, the diagnosis is still in doubt and the surgeon has to proceed to marker wire localization diagnostic biopsy. At this operation the surgeon removes only a small piece of tissue through a short incision (Figure 65); if the lesion proves to be benign, the woman should be left with no significant cosmetic defect. To achieve this, the surgeon needs to be able to take the shortest approach directly to the tip of the wire and not have to follow the wire down through a considerable length of breast tissue. It follows that the surgeon needs to be able to palpate the area in which the tip of the wire lies, preferably before he has cut the skin. A marker-wire set which enables the surgeon to do this has been designed (the Nottingham Needle) (Figure 66). The radiologist places the wire within the lesion (Figure 67), the surgeon removes a small amount of tissue - the recommended upper limit is 20 g but usually a smaller piece is removed (Figure 68). A specimen X-ray is taken as shown in Figure 68, to confirm that the lesion has been removed.

If the surgeon is carrying out a marker wire localization operation for therapeutic reasons, the preoperative diagnosis of cancer having been made by cytology, a considerably larger piece of tissue is removed and a specimen X-ray is taken to ensure that the impalpable lesion has been removed and appears clear from the circumferential margins (Figure 69). In the histology laboratory, the specimen X-ray is further used to determine which block should be examined for the presence of the lesion (Figure 70). The distribution of cancers found in the first round of screening (the prevalent screen) is shown in Figure 71. Approximately a quarter of the cancers are carcinoma in situ; approximately a quarter are those with an excellent prognosis as shown by the Nottingham Prognosis Index and may be considered cured of breast cancer; approximately a quarter are those with a good prognosis with a high likelihood of survival at 20 years post-operation and only a quarter are those with only a moderate or poor prognosis. This contrasts with the distribution (Figure 72) in symptomatic (referred) cancers; far more screen detected cancers are in good prognostic groups and very few have a poor prognosis. The survival graph of tumors in the excellent prognostic group in the last 10 years in Nottingham is seen in Figure 73, by nine years the cause specific mortality is less than 5%.

Figure 55

Assessment. About 4% of women are recalled for assessment following their screening examination. Assessment consists of further imaging, physical examination and cytological examination, carried out by a multidisciplinary team. Approximately 1% of women screened will require surgery and the majority of these will be found to have breast cancer. A definite diagnosis of cancer is made before surgery in most cases, allowing them to go straight to definitive treatment.

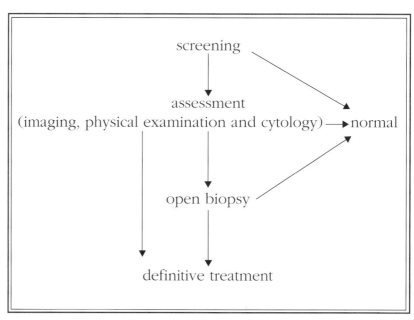

Figure 56

Microcalcification. This magnification mammogram demonstrates calcification. Microcalcification is a very common mammographic finding. In the vast majority of cases it is benign. Benign calcifications are typically punctate, diffusely distributed and associated with lobular cystic change. Malignant calcifications tend to show pleomorphism and are inclined to show a ductal distribution.

Microcalcifications in the figure below show elongated rod and Y-shaped forms and have a positive predictive value for malignancy of about 85%. They are most often due to comedo sub-type DCIS. Other suspicious microcalcifications, such as granular calcifications of variable density and size, have a positive predictive value of malignancy of approximately 35%.

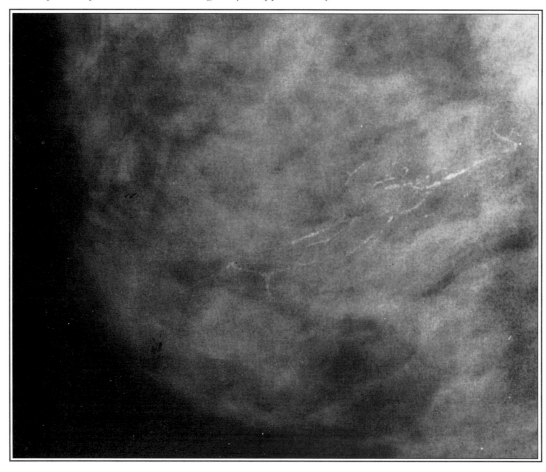

Figure 57

Histological section of ductal carcinoma in situ of the breast. This photomicrograph shows a breast duct filled by a population of large pleomorphic cells. These cells are confined within the basement membrane of the duct and show no evidence of infiltration to adjacent breast tissues.

The cells in the center of the duct space have become necrotic. Such areas of necrosis frequently undergo calcification which can be detected mammographically.

In well differentiated forms of ductal carcinoma in situ, glandular structures can be produced by the tumor cells. The secretions within these glandular spaces can also undergo calcification which may be detectable mammographically.

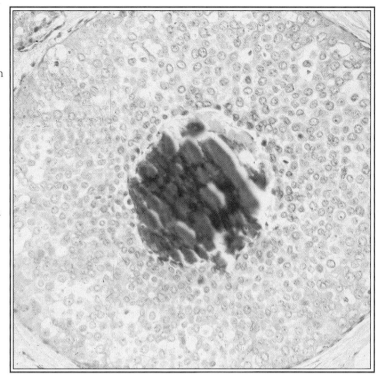

Figure 58

Impalpable breast lesions. This mammogram shows a small stellate mass in the right upper outer quadrant which proved to be a carcinoma. Diagnosis of impalpable lesions detected at screening is with image guided FNA. FNA is most easily performed under ultrasound guidance and the majority of impalpable suspicious masses can be visualized using this technique. Ultrasound can also be used to localize lesions for excision biopsy.

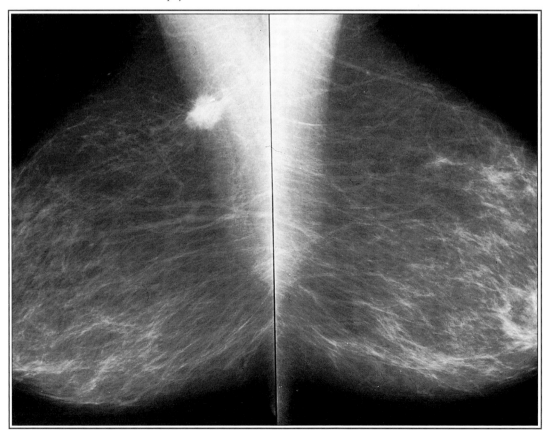

Figure 59

Histological section of an invasive adenocarcinoma of tubular type. This is an example of a 'special type' of breast carcinoma. Tumors in this group have an extremely good long-term prognosis. In the tubular type the tumor cells are well differentiated and form tubular or glandular structures very similar to the acinar glands within the normal terminal duct lobulae.

This particular special type of breast cancer is found more commonly in mammographic screening programs.

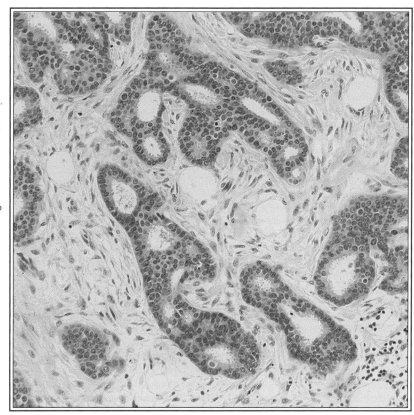

Figure 60

Stereotactic device. A stereotactic device demonstrating the position of the machine for taking the two images at 30 degrees apart. The exact location of the mammographically-detected abnormality is calculated using these images.

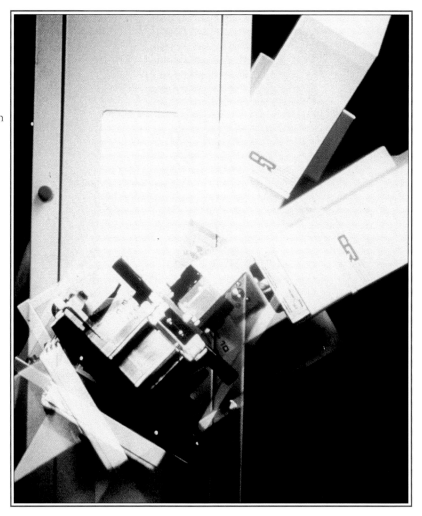

Figure 61

Image guided FNA. Stereotactically guided FNA. The use of sampling using five or more needle passes has increased our adequacy rate to more than 85%. The procedure is normally well tolerated if local anesthetic is used. Stereotactic FNA can be accurate to within a millimeter.

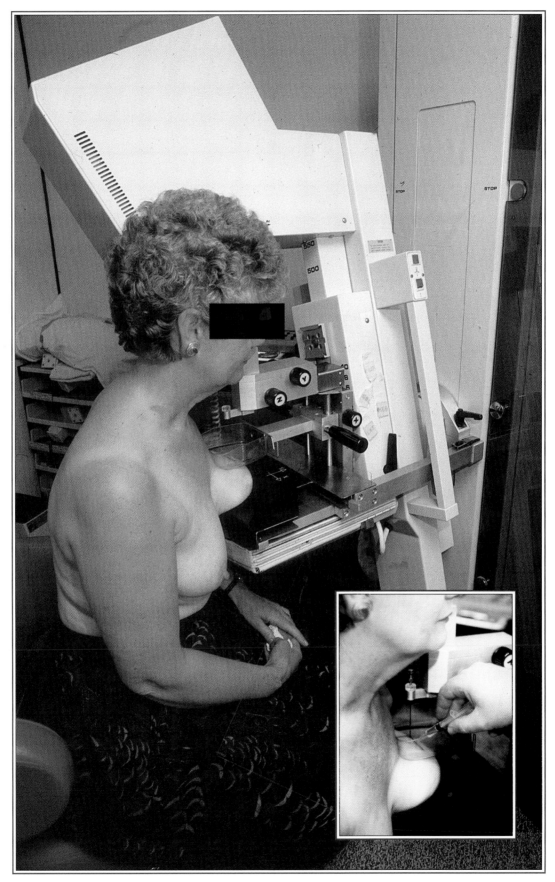

Figure 62

Image guided FNA. This image shows the correct position of the needle tip within an ill-defined mass. Films should always be performed to confirm the accurate localization of either a needle for FNA or placement of a marker wire.

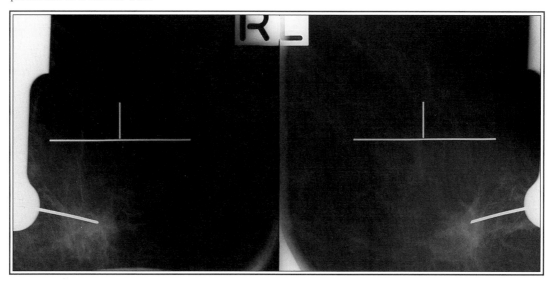

Figure 63

Architectural distortion. Localized areas of architectural distortion in a stellate pattern are common diagnostic problems in the interpretation of screening mammograms.

Differential diagnosis of this appearance is between a radial scar/complex sclerosing lesion and a carcinoma, typically of the tubular type. This type of stellate lesion is usually impalpable.

It may be visible on ultrasound, but its ultrasound features are not helpful in differentiating benign from malignant processes. Radial scars are said not to have a central mass, and to show architectural distortion only in one plane; however, these distinguishing features are unreliable and all such lesions should be excised. If visible on ultrasound, this technique can be used for sampling and localization. The lesion here proved to be a radial scar.

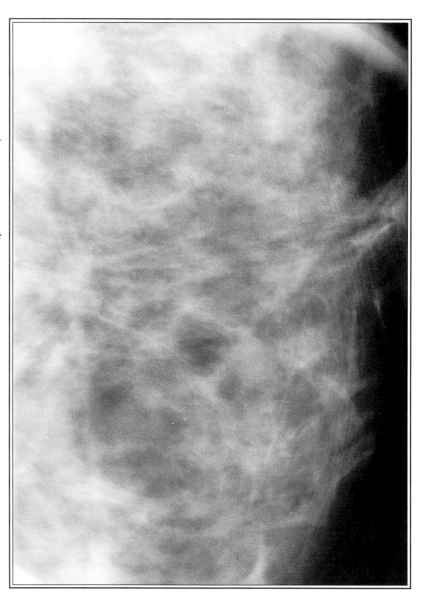

Figure 64

Histological section of radial scar. Radial scars have a stellate configuration with radiating arms containing ductal or acinar structures.

In their sclerotic centers they are composed of densely hyalinized and collagenous stromal tissue which entraps glandular structures, as shown in this illustration. Their appearance is similar to the 'crab' shape seen in many breast cancers (Figure 30) which may lead to misdiagnosis of carcinoma mammographically.

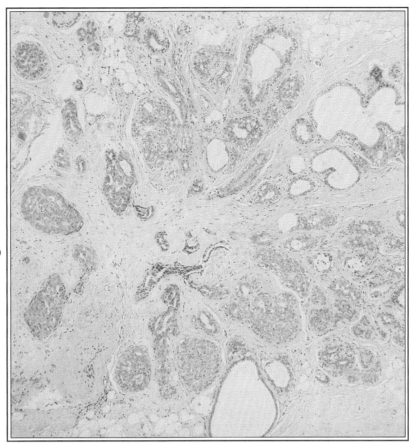

Figure 65

Biopsy. Incision for removal of a small piece of breast tissue containing an impalpable lesion at marker wire localization biopsy.

It can be seen that the incision is small and there is no visible defect in the breast tissue because only a small piece has been removed. On this occasion, it was possible to place the incision around the areola. The scar will be invisible 18 months to 2 years after operation.

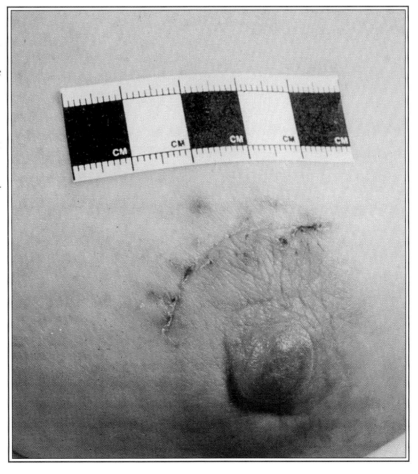

Figure 66

The Nottingham marker wire localization set. This is used to enable the surgeon to palpate the area in which the tip of the marker wire lies.

The wire may be inserted under ultrasound guidance or using the technique described in Figure 61. When the patient comes to the operating theater, a cannula is placed over the marker wire and led down to the tip of the wire.

The surgeon may then feel the tip of the cannula through the skin and is able to make a small incision directly over the tip and excise only the tissue at the tip of the needle.

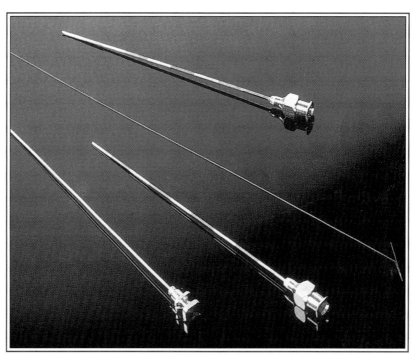

Figure 67

Localization of impalpable breast lesions. The mammogram shows localization of an impalpable mass using the Nottingham lesion location device. This procedure is quick and easy to perform, particularly using ultrasound guidance.

Stereotactic guidance should be used if the lesion is ultrasonically occult.

For guiding complete excision of an area of microcalcification, two wires may be inserted, marking the outer limits of the area for excision.

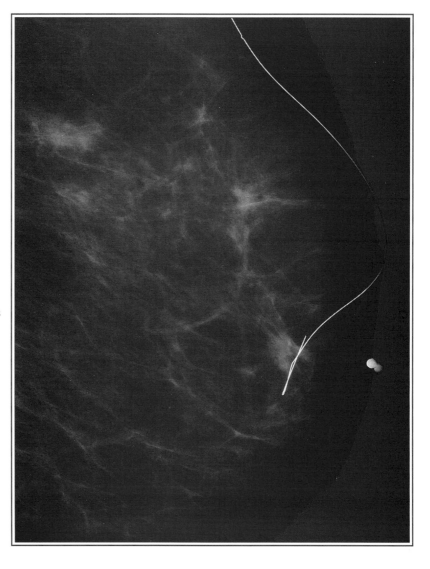

Figure 68

Specimen X-ray of a lesion removed for diagnostic purposes. The amount of breast tissue removed is small: this biopsy weighed around 12g. There is no attempt to remove an extra margin around the tissue because a diagnosis has not yet been made. Should this lesion contain a cancer it will be necessary to carry out a second operation for a much wider excision and also to biopsy the lymph nodes.

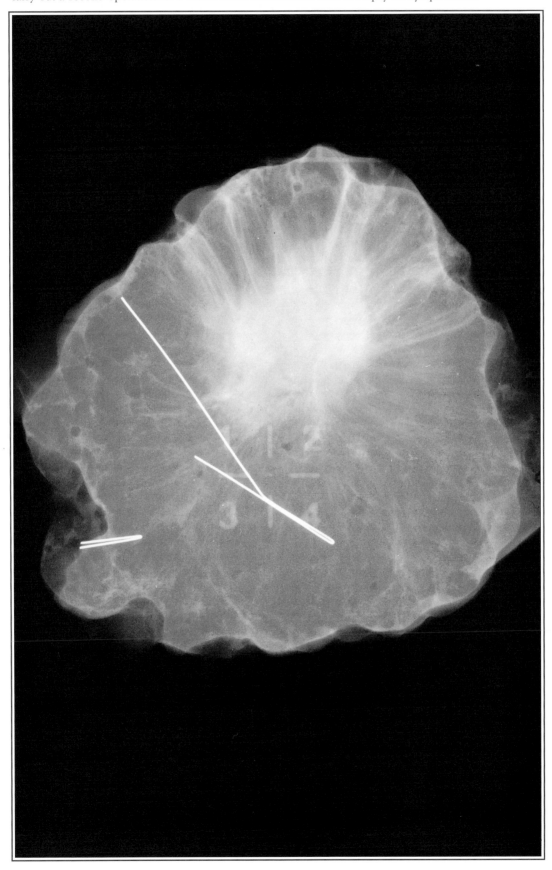

Figure 69

Excision of an impalpable breast cancer. The diagnosis has already been made by cytology. A much larger piece of tissue (weighing around 70g) than the piece in Figure 68 has been removed in an attempt to gain clear margins around the tumor. Although these margins appear to be sufficiently far from the tumor for this to be acceptable, the definitive check will be made at histology.

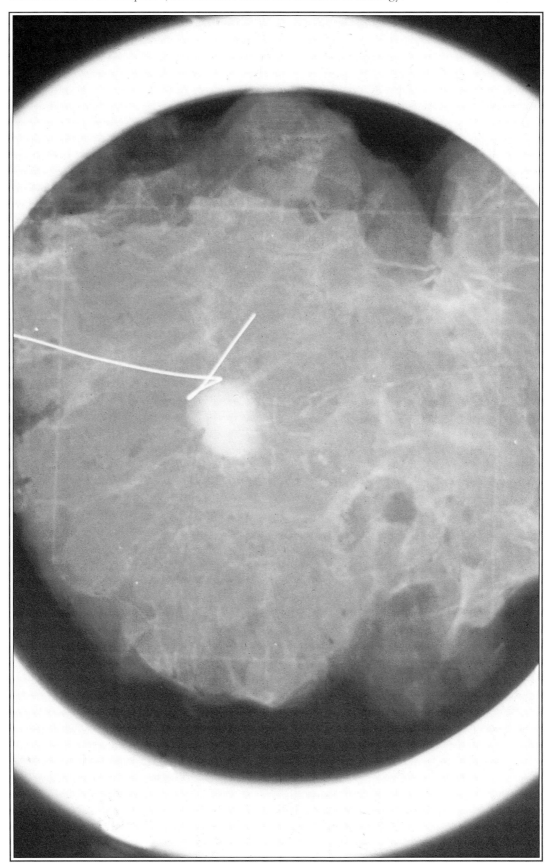

Figure 70

Specimen X-ray. X-ray is used to examine excised tissue to identify the block most likely to contain the lesion for the histologist to examine.

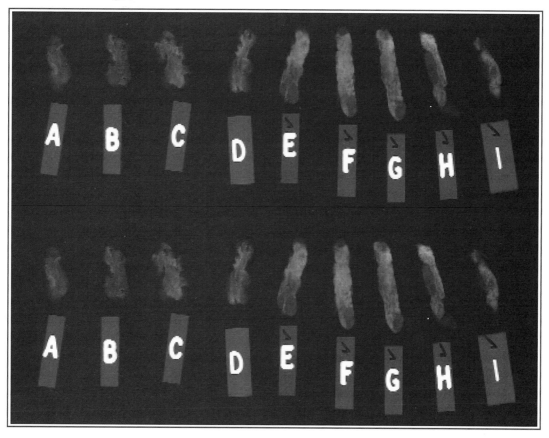

Figure 71

The presentation of cancers detected at breast cancer screening according to prognostic group. A quarter of the cancers present as ductal carcinoma in situ, a quarter as excellent prognosis invasive, a quarter in the good prognostic group, and only a quarter in the moderate and poor prognostic groups (see legend to Figure 54).

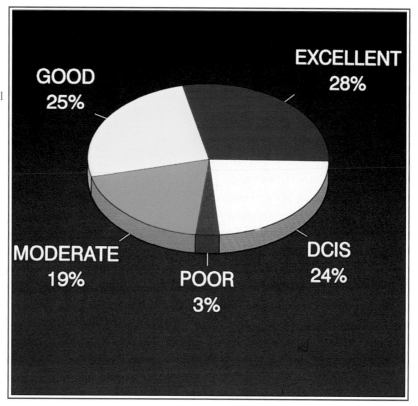

Figure 72

GP referral. To contrast with Figure 71, this is the presentation of cancer patients referred by their general practitioners to the symptomatic clinic. Far fewer than in the screen detected group are seen in the excellent prognostic group and far more in the poor prognostic group.

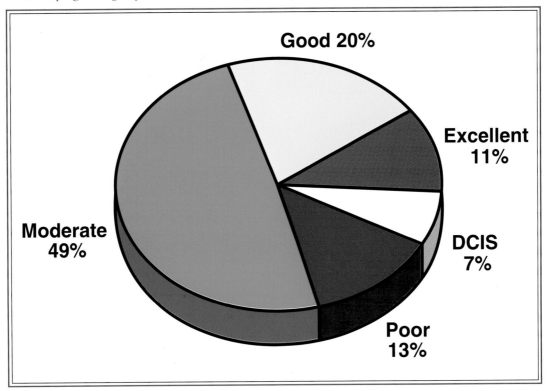

Figure 73

The long-term survival of patients with tumors sized 2 cm or less, node negative on biopsy, histology grade 1.
As seen in Figure 72, around 30% of the cancers detected at breast cancer screening fall into this group (EPG).

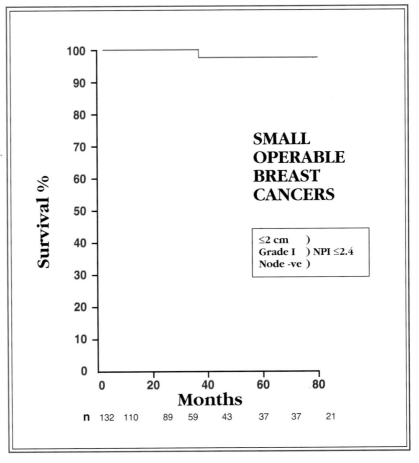

SECTION 6

LOCAL AND REGIONAL PROBLEMS

SECTION 6

LOCAL AND REGIONAL PROBLEMS

In contrast to the excellent outlook for many of the cancers found at breast cancer screening, a number of cancers still present symptomatically at a locally advanced stage (Figures 74 & 75). These cancers have a generally poor outlook - only some 30% of patients presenting at this stage are still alive five years later. They seem to present in two ways (1) as very aggressive tumors suddenly showing as marked oedema (peau d'orange) of the breast, as seen in Figure 74; and (2) as a more indolent type of tumor, which causes scarring and contracture of the breast as shown in Figure 75 or an indolent ulcer. The first type of presentation indicates a tumor that has become extensive without forming a lump in the breast and only presents when the whole breast has its lymphatic channels blocked. Such an appearence is sometimes known as 'inflammatory cancer'. The second type of presentation is more often seen in elderly women and is less aggressive. Both forms - but especially the former - may be difficult to control locally. Radiotherapy and/or hormonal therapy (Figures 76 & 77) may be initially successful in holding back the tumor.

LOCAL RECURRENCE AFTER MASTECTOMY

Local recurrence in the mastectomy flaps is seen in three forms. The first is a single subcutaneous or intracutaneous spot, which is usually successfully treated by excision under local anesthetic. This appears to result from a small amount of tumor being left behind by the surgeon and reflects the fact that surgery is much less radical than in previous eras. Multiple spot recurrence (Figure 78) and extensive intralymphatic intradermal spread, as shown in Figure 79, are indications of a much more aggressive biological type of disease and particularly occur in the presence of grade III tumors with vascular invasion (Figure 48). Vascular invasion is a predisposing factor to local recurrence, both after breast conservation (see above) and after mastectomy. Local recurrence following mastectomy is, to some extent, preventable by prophylactic flap irradiation. Patients who have grade III primary tumors with vascular invasion have a high chance of local recurrence and should have such prophylaxis. Once it has occurred, local recurrence may necessitate extensive surgery (Figure 80).

REGIONAL RECURRENCE

Metastases to regional lymph nodes (Figure 81) are seen in a number of patients in the follow-up of primary breast cancer. Without prophylactic irradiation or total axillary clearance, around one third of patients subsequently develop palpable metastatic lymph nodes in the axilla. With prophylactic irradiation or complete dissection, the proportion is closer to 10%. However, this means that were prophylactic irradiation to be given to all patients, some 70% would be receiving it unnecessarily, since they would either never develop nodal recurrence even without such irradiation or would have developed it despite irradiation. Therefore, as for the prevention of local recurrence (above), at our center, prophylactic irradiation is reserved for the selected group most at risk of developing nodal recurrence: that is the patients who have a positive lymph node on biopsy at operation and have an aggressive primary tumor (grade III).

Involvement of the internal mammary nodes may occasionally give rise to problems in follow-up (Figure 82).

Two trials carried out in the 1970s, the NSABP trial in the USA and the CRC trial the UK, showed that prophylactic node dissection or irradiation does not affect survival. This is because the primary route of spread is through the blood stream. Whether the patient subsequently dies from breast cancer depends upon whether or not distant metastases are present at the time of diagnosis of the primary cancer.

Figure 74

Advanced primary breast cancer. Considerable skin oedema (peau d'orange) can be seen. There is also retraction of the nipple.

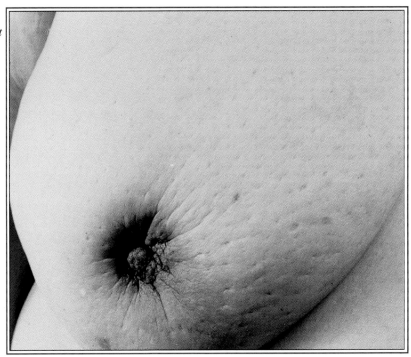

Figure 75

Advanced primary breast cancer. Shrinkage of the left breast with skin attachment is seen.

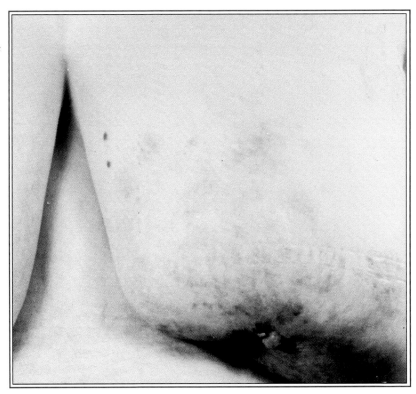

Figure 76

Advanced primary tumor before treatment.

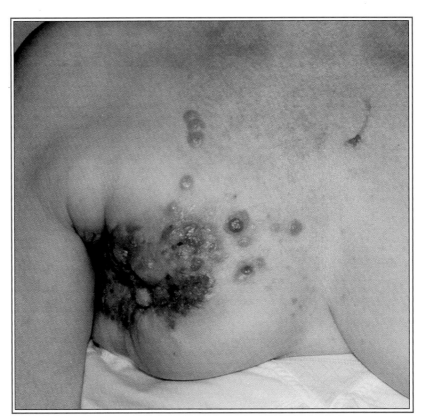

Figure 77

Advanced primary tumor previously shown in Figure 76 which has improved after treatment with Tamoxifen. Tamoxifen may control the tumor for a limited length of time, after which it returns in the treated breast.

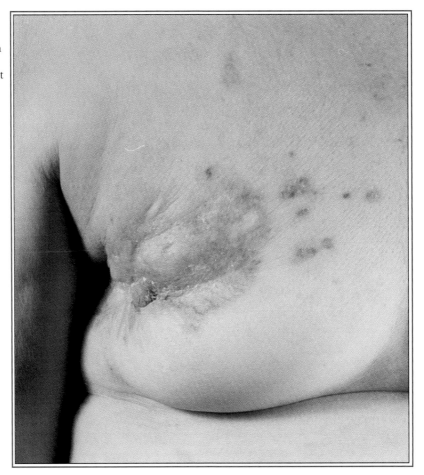

Figure 78

Skin recurrence in the mastectomy flaps, multiple spot type.

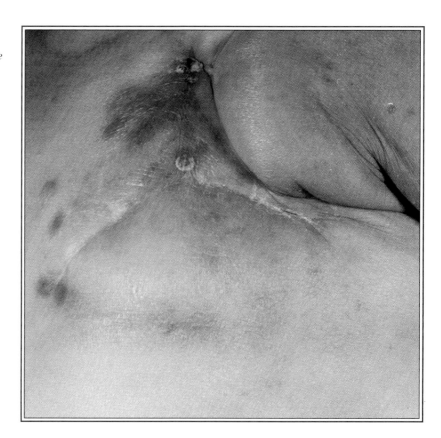

Figure 79

Recurrence in the mastectomy flaps extending round to the back. This intradermal lymphatic spread is often impossible to control by local means, necessitating systemic therapies. However. these are usually unsuccessful.

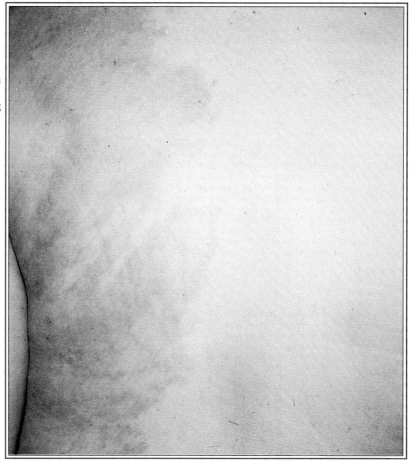

Figure 80

A woman who has undergone an *Omental flap* after very wide excision of locally recurrent breast cancer, followed by mobilizing the omentum to cover the area; split skin grafts are placed on the omentum.

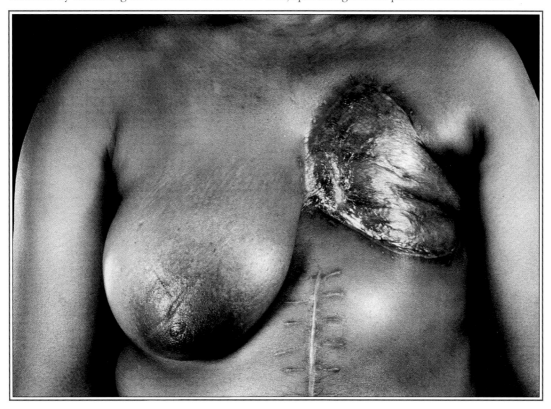

Figure 81

Axillary lymph node removed for staging purposes from a patient with an invasive adenocarcinoma of the breast. This node shows extensive replacement of its normal structure by metastatic tumor cells identical to those seen in the primary breast tumor. In this illustration an area of normal lymph node with peripheral sinus can be identified adjacent to the carcinoma deposit.

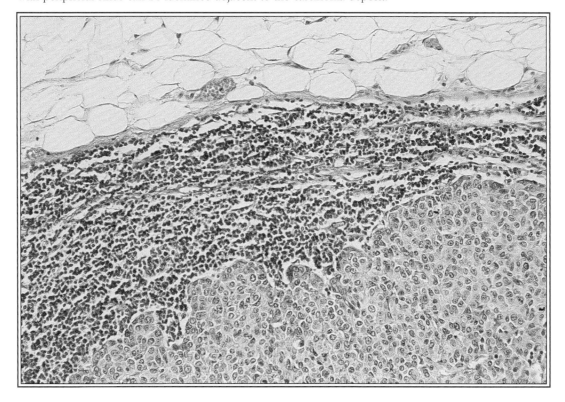

Figure 82

Metastasis in an internal mammary node that has grown and is invading through the skin.

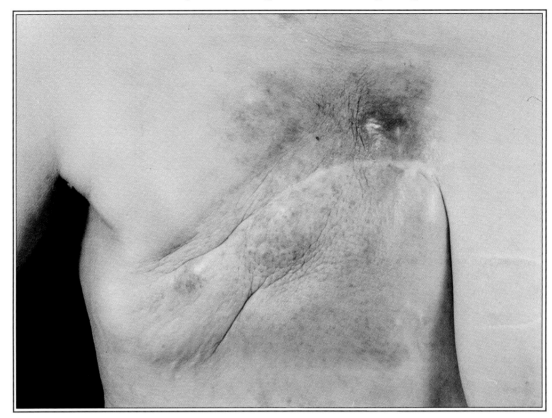

SECTION 7

DISTANT METASTASES

SECTION 7

DISTANT METASTASES

The distribution of breast cancer metastases is similar to that of any cancer spreading through the systemic, rather than the portal, circulation. The principle site of metastasis is in the bone (Figures 83-85). Particular problems associated with bone metastases are the pain they cause, and bony destruction which may give rise to fracture of long bones (Figure 86) or to collapse of the vertebral column and paraplegia. Pain control may be achieved with radiotherapy, but the structural problems require orthopedic stabilization (Figure 87).

Another symptom of metastasis may be breathlessness, most often caused by pleural effusion (Figure 88). This probably arises as a result of lymphatic spread from the primary tumor, as it is more likely to occur with large primary tumors and appears ipsilateral to the primary tumor. Other metastatic manifestations are solid intrapulmonary metastases (Figure 89) and lymphangitis carcinomatosa of the lung (Figure 88), which is often difficult to recognize on X-ray.

Pleural effusion requires drainage and pleurodesis to prevent recurrence. Breathlessness due to intrapulmonary metastases or lymphangitis requires aggressive chemotherapy to relieve the symptoms. Liver metastases (Figures 90 & 91) and CNS metastases (Figure 92) may also occur and are indication of a very poor outlook.

TREATMENT OF SYSTEMIC METASTASES

As briefly referred to above, treatment of systemic metastases is often symptomatically led. Attempts to slow down their growth by hormonal means or by using chemotherapy may be made. The best outcome is achieved when a tumor is responsive to hormones; this may be predicted estrogen receptor positivity of the primary tumor (Figure 53). The usual first time endocrine therapy for post-menopausal women is to use the estrogen blocking agent, Tamoxifen. Pre-menopausal women may also have their ovarian function blocked, perhaps medically using LH-RH agonists.

Figure 83

Bony metastases. This radiograph of the pelvis shows multiple ill-defined areas of sclerosis, indicating osteoblastic metastases. Bony metastases from breast carcinoma may be lytic, sclerotic or show a mixed pattern. Radiographs are essential in assessing response or progression of disease, but are not as sensitive as scintigraphy or MR imaging in the detection of bony metastases.

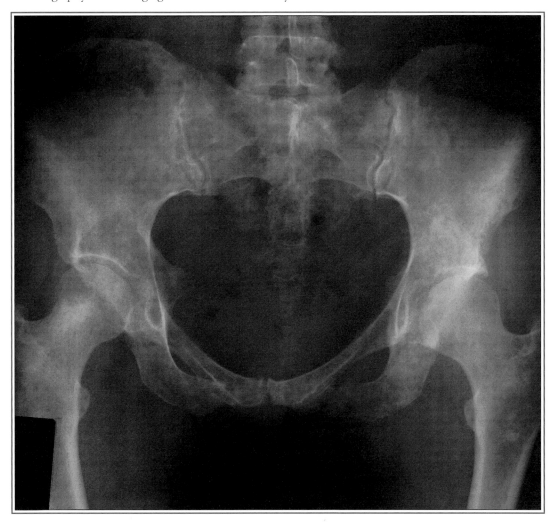

Figure 84

Bony metastases. MR imaging is exquisitely sensitive to metastatic involvement of bone marrow. It is also useful for the evaluation of response of bone metastases to treatment. Changes in signal characteristics on MR occur very early with treatment either with chemotherapy or with radiotherapy and can be used to assess response to treatment. MR also has the advantage over skeletal scintigraphy of providing excellent anatomical detail. In the spine this is useful for showing potential and actual spinal cord compression.

The illustration is of a T1 weighted image showing areas of reduced signal within the L4 and L5 vertebral bodies, indicating metastatic involvement.

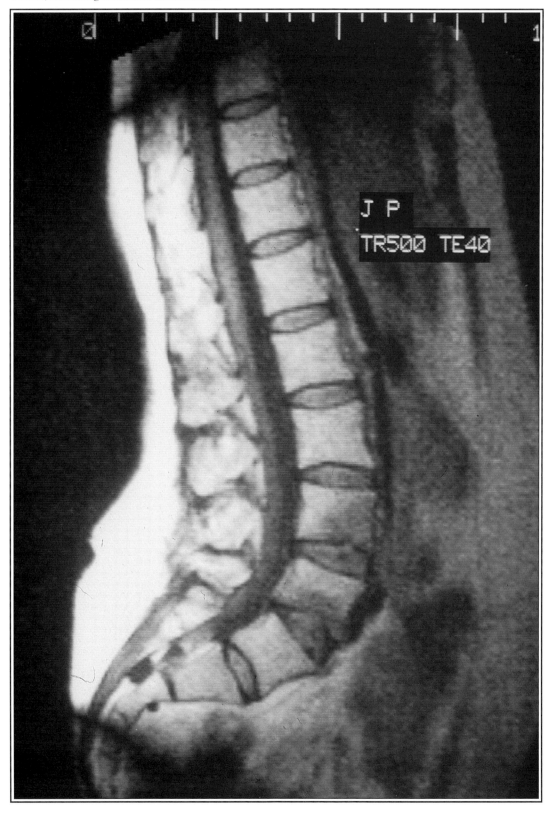

Figure 85

Bony metastases.
Skeletal scintigraphy is
a useful investigation in
terms of demonstrating
bony involvement with
metastatic disease. It is
more sensitive than
plain film radiology.
This skeletal scintigram
demonstrates increased
photon activity in the
ribs, shoulder, spine
and pelvis, representing
metastatic deposits.

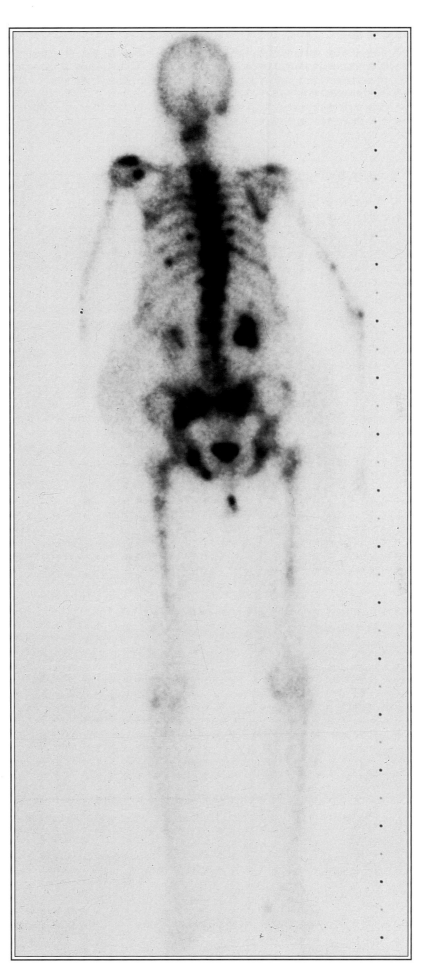

Figure 86

Pathological fracture of the shaft of the humerus.

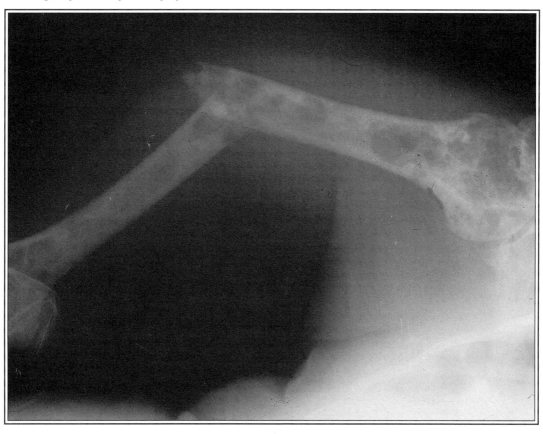

Figure 87

Prosthetic hip replacement following a pathological fracture of the right femoral neck.

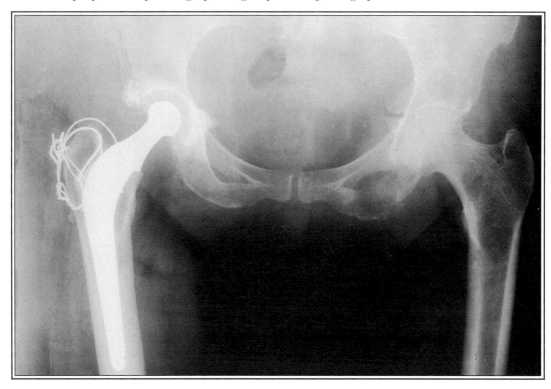

Figure 88

Pleural metastases and lymphangitis. This chest radiograph shows fine linear shadowing radiating from the left hilum, indicating lymphangitis carcinomatosa. This is associated with a malignant pleural effusion on the left side.

Pleural metastases are commonly seen in breast cancer and may present radiologically as a pleural effusion with no other features; However, lobulated pleural masses are also sometimes demonstrated.

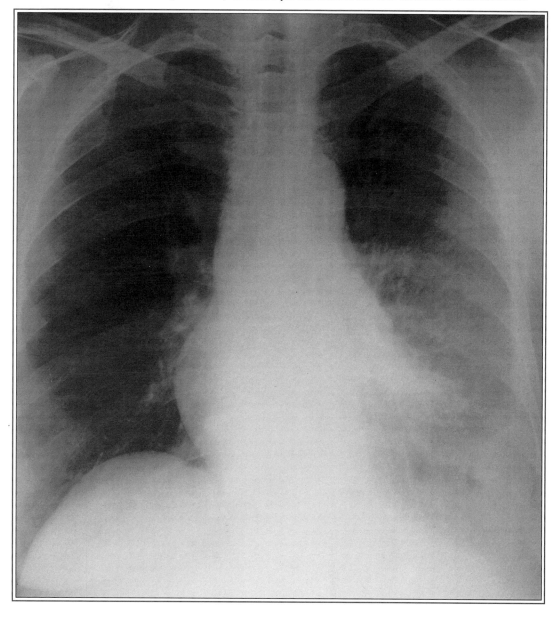

Figure 89

Pulmonary metastases. This chest radiograph shows multiple intrapulmonary masses bilaterally, indicating widespread pulmonary metastases.

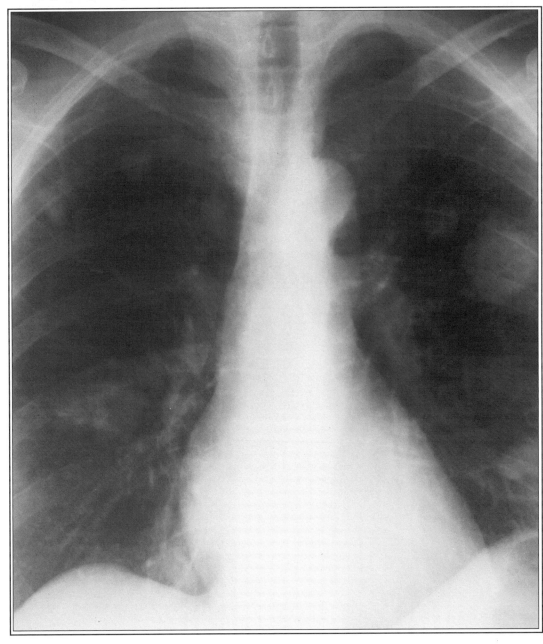

Figure 90

Liver metastases.
The simplest and most cost-effective way to assess the liver in patients with possible symptoms of advanced breast cancer is to perform ultrasound. The image below shows clear evidence of metastatic disease from breast cancer. Lesions are demonstrated as discreet rounded hypoechoic or hyperechoic masses. Occasionally, liver metastases produce a more diffuse picture of variable liver echogenicity.

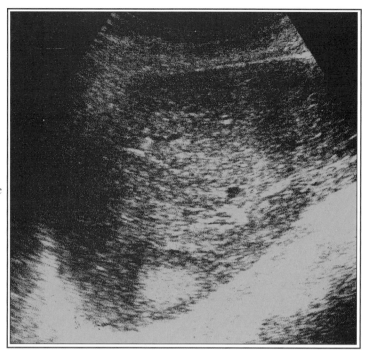

Figure 91

Liver metastases.
CT scanning of the liver is more sensitive than ultrasound in the demonstration of liver metastases.

The majority of metastases are demonstrated as areas of lower attenuation than surrounding liver tissue.

The use of intravenous contrast marginally increases the sensitivity of CT scanning in the demonstration of metastases. This image demonstrates a rib metastasis as well as liver metastases.

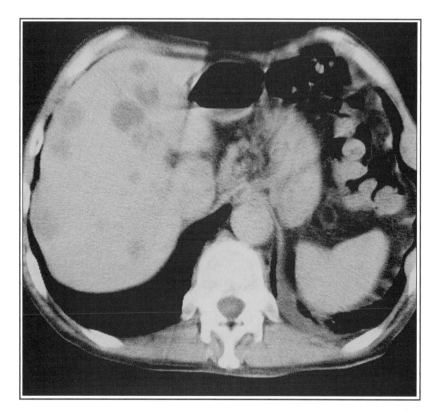

Figure 92

Contrast enhanced brain CT demonstrating multiple, ring enhancing cerebral metastases. The large metastasis in the right hemisphere shows considerable surrounding oedema.

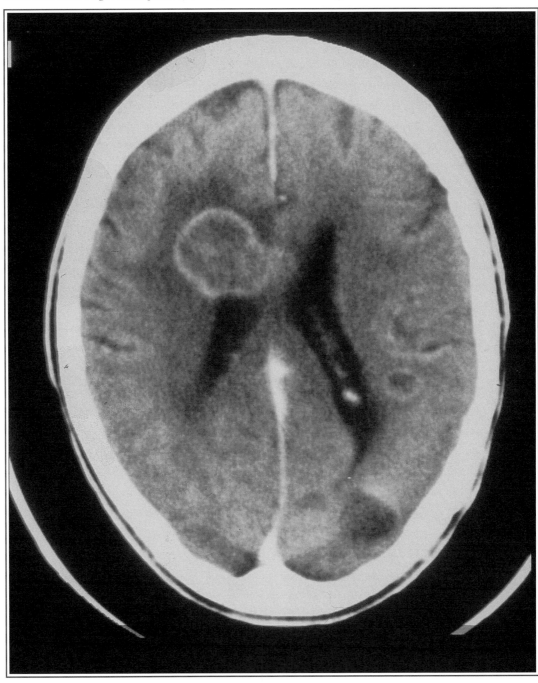

SECTION 8

PHYLLODES TUMOR

SECTION 8

PHYLLODES TUMOR

A phyllodes tumor often presents as a very large lump in the breast. The diagnosis is suggested by the observation that there is no skin or deep attachment, despite the tumor's considerable size (Figure 93). The name phyllodes is derived from the Greek for 'leaf' and comes about because of the tumor's leaf-like appearance when cut across (Figure 94). Such tumors tend to be large at presentation because, when small, they feel much like the surrounding normal tissue. Occasionally, impalpable phyllodes tumours as large as 3 cm are detected at mammographic screening (Figures 95 & 96). Phyllodes tumors are essentially benign (Figure 97), although rare examples are sarcomatous.

Figure 93

Phyllodes tumor of the breast. Although there is a very large tumor in the breast, there is no skin attachment, ulceration or deep attachment.

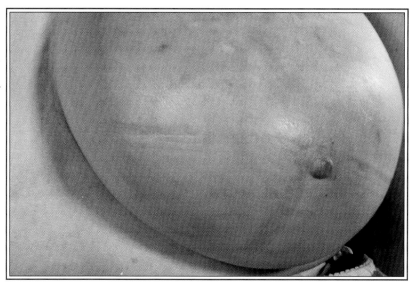

Figure 94

The cut surface of a phyllodes tumor, showing the leaf-like structure.

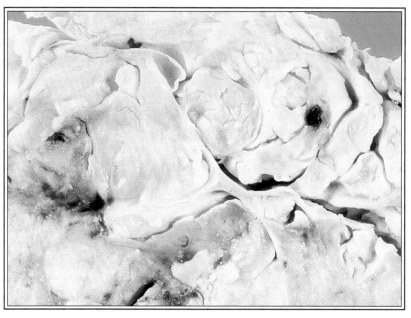

Figure 95

Phyllodes tumor.
Phyllodes tumors present
mammographically
as well-defined masses
which may be very large.

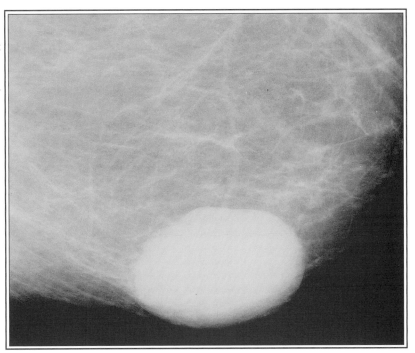

Figure 96

Phyllodes tumor.
Ultrasound of phyllodes
tumors show a solid
homogeneous tumor
with well-defined
margins. There may be
distal acoustic
enhancement.

In about 50% of cases
there are discrete areas
of increased
echogenicity within the
tumor and occasionally
leaf-like highly echogenic
septations are
demonstrated, as shown.

This appearance is
virtually pathognomonic
for a phyllodes tumor.

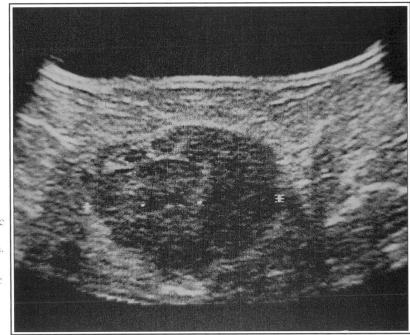

Figure 97

Phyllodes tumor of the breast. Phyllodes tumors have components similar to fibroadenomas, that is, epithelial glandular tissue and stromal tissue.

They differ in the degree of stromal proliferation, and the presence of atypia of the stromal cells. Histological examination, as shown in this illustration, confirms a combination of epithelial and stromal tissue. The stroma shows cellular atypia and pleomorphism.

Phyllodes tumors can be classified as benign, borderline or malignant on the basis of the proportion of epithelial to stromal tissue, the degree of atypia within the stroma, and infiltration into the adjacent breast tissue.

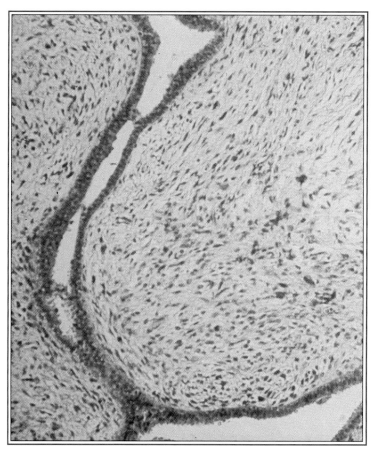

Figure 98

Mondor's syndrome. The line of the thrombosed vein is clearly seen; typically, it lies down the lateral side of the breast.

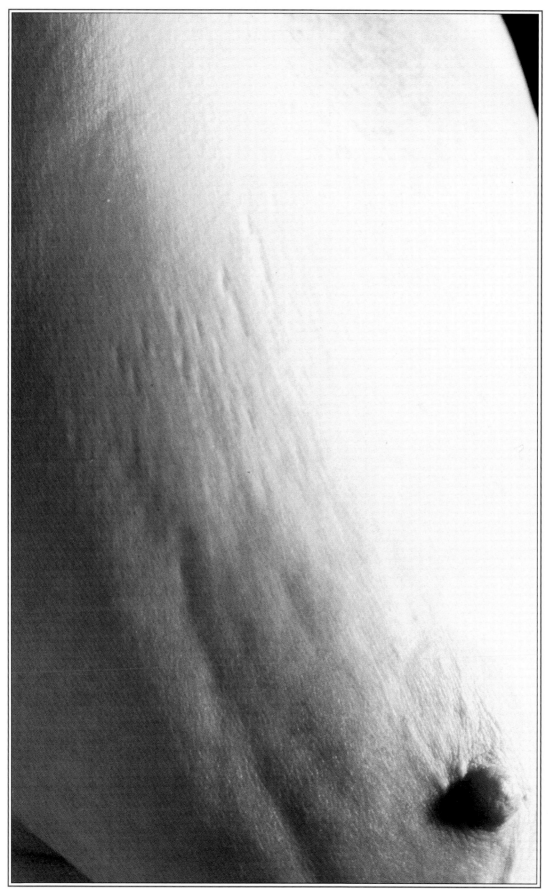

SECTION 9

RARE PROBLEMS

SECTION 9

RARE PROBLEMS

Mondor's syndrome

Mondor's syndrome (Figure 98) is thrombosis of a vein, usually down the lateral side of the breast. Its appearance, particularly at the lower end, includes a small area of skin tether that may cause alarm. It is easily diagnosed because the thrombosed vein is seen throughout the length of the breast and may be palpated by rolling it underneath the finger, when it is felt as a cord within the breast.

Juvenile fibroadenomatosis

Juvenile fibroadenomatosis is often felt as a very large lump within the breast of a woman around the age of 20. It has a somewhat irregular edge. Despite its alarming feel, this lesion is entirely benign, although it may require removal for cosmetic reasons.

Adenosis of pregnancy

In pregnancy, a breast duct system may become very firm to the feel and present as a symmetrical lump around 4-6 cm in diameter. Needle histological biopsy reveals only breast tissue with pregnancy changes.

Male breast cancer (Figure 99)

Male breast cancer is rarely seen. Most breast lumps in men are symmetrically located under the nipple and are simply gynecomastia. Occasionally, more irregular lumps located eccentrically are seen and must be investigated as possible cancers.

Figure 99

A breast cancer presenting as Paget's disease of the nipple in a male.

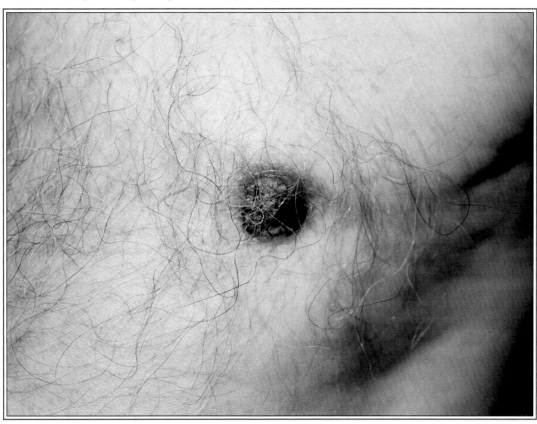

Figure 100

The Nottingham Breast Diagnostic Team. Although the named authors produced the illustrations at the demand of our Editor, the Atlas represents the work of the whole Nottingham Diagnostic Team pictured here.

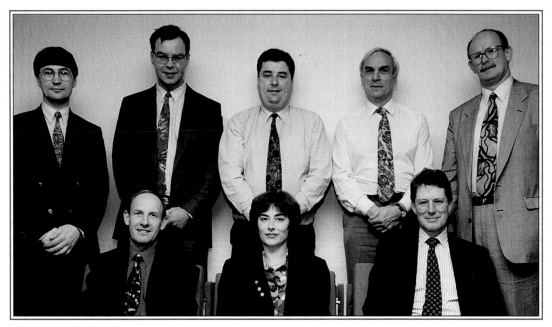

Standing: John Robertson, Andy Evans, Mark Sibbering, Roger Blamey, Robin Wilson.
Sitting: Chris Elston, Lindsey Yeoman, Ian Ellis.

POSTSCRIPT

POSTSCRIPT

The diagnosis and management of breast disease rely on traditional principals of good elicitation of physical signs and careful use and good interpretation of investigative techniques. We have tried to illustrate many of these in this Atlas. We hope it will prove useful to medical and paramedical staff of all levels who wish to gain straightforward knowledge of breast disease.

Although an appreciation of physical signs, skill in the taking and reading of X-rays, and an understanding of the problems of a woman with advanced breast cancer can only be gained by attendance at specialist breast clinics, this book will prompt those visiting clinics to search out the various problems illustrated.